Renal Transplantation

General Editor, Wolfe Surgical Atlases:
William F. Walker, DSc, ChM, FRCS (Edin. and
England), FRS (Edin.).

Single Surgical Procedures 13

A Colour Atlas of

Renal Transplantation

Roy Y. Calne
MA, MS, FRCS, FRS
Professor of Surgery,
Department of Surgery,
University of Cambridge

Wolfe Medical Publications Ltd

Published by Wolfe Medical Publications Ltd, 1984
Printed by Royal Smeets Offset b.v.,
Weert, Netherlands
ISBN 0 7234 1024 0

This book is one of the titles in the series of
Wolfe Single Surgical Procedures, a series which
will eventually cover some 200 titles.
   If you wish to be kept informed of new
additions to the series and receive details of our
other titles, please write to
Wolfe Medical Publications Ltd, Wolfe House,
3 Conway Street, London W1P 6HE.

**A few of the other titles in print and in preparation
in the Single Surgical Procedures series**

Parotidectomy
Traditional Meniscectomy
*Inguinal Hernias & Hydroceles in Infants and
   Children*
*Surgery for Pancreatic & Associated
   Carcinomata*
Subtotal Thyroidectomy
Boari Bladder-Flap Procedure
Treatment of Carpal Tunnel Syndrome
Anterior Resection of Rectum

Seromyotomy for Chronic Duodenal Ulcer
Resection of Aortic Aneurysm
Modified Radical Mastectomy
Total Gastrectomy
Ileo-Rectal Anastomosis
Pre-Prosthetic Oral Surgery
Surgery for Undescended Testes
Techniques of Nerve Grafting and Repair
Surgery for Dupuytren's Contracture
Athrodesis of the Ankle
Surgery for Congenital Dislocation of the Hip
Common Operations of the Foot
Femoral and Tibial Osteotomy
Maxillo-Facial Traumatology
Surgery for Chondromalacia Patellae
Stabilisation for Extensive Spinal Injury
Spondylolisthesis
Laminectomy
Gall Bladder Cholecystectomy
Repair of Prolapsed Rectum
Proctocolectomy
Resection of Oesophagus
Splenectomy
Thyroid Lobectomy
Hirschprung's Disease
Extra-cranial and Intra-cranial Anastomosis
Anterior Nephrectomy
Bladder Augmentation
Caecocystoplasty
Hiatus Hernia
Total Gastrectomy
Billroth 1 Gastrectomy
Billroth 2 Gastrectomy
Abdominal Incisions
Thoracotomy
Chronic Pancreatitis Operation
Surgery for Strictures in Common Bile Duct
Biliary Enteric Anastomosis
Partial Hepatectomy
Splenectomy
Right Hemicolectomy
Appendicectomy
Incisional Hernia
Lung Lobectomy
Lung Removal
Gastric Reconstruction
Surgery for Lymphoedema
Kidney Transplants
Liver Transplant
Pancreas Transplant
Dialysis Techniques

Surgery for Thoracic Outlet
Haemorrhoids
Abdominoperineal Resection of Rectum
Rectosigmoid Resection
*Non-resectional Surgery for Multiple Bowel
   Stenosis*
Surgery for Anorectal Incontinence
Carotid Surgery
Craniotomy
Parathyroidectomy
Arterial Injuries
Arterial Bypass Grafts in Leg
Visceral Vascular Occlusion
Varicose Veins under Local Anaesthesia
Aortofemoral Bypass
Aortoiliac Disobliteration
Technique of Small Vessel Repair
Technique of Nerve Grafting and Repair
Microsurgery Techniques
Reimplantation of Ureters
Pyloric Stenosis in Children
Cleft Palate Surgery
Anorectal Malformation
Amputations of the Lower Limb
Anterolateral Decompression
Spinal Fusion
Scoliosis
Spinal Fusion for Low Back Pain
Anterior Fusion of Cervical Spine
Recurrent Dislocation of Shoulder
Joint Replacement of Elbow
Joint Replacement of Wrist and Hand
Operative Fixation of Fractures of the Forearm
Joint Replacement at the Hip
Joint Replacement at the Knee
Arthrodesis of the Knee
Triple Arthrodesis
Discogram Surgery – Lumbar Disc
Amputations of the Upper Limb and Hand
Plastering Techniques
*Operations for Peripheral Nerve
Compression Syndromes*
*Techniques of Tendon Transfer in the Upper
   Limb*
Arthrodesis of the Wrist
Reconstructive Procedures of the Thumb
Flexor Tendon Repair and Grafting
Minor Operative Procedures
Technique of Arthroscopy of the Knee
*Management of Fresh Ligamentous Injuries
   of the Knee*

Contents

Introduction

The object of renal transplantation is to provide the recipient suffering from irrecoverable renal failure with an allografted vascularised kidney that will function and maintain him in good health for a long period. The selection and preparation of recipients, their postoperative monitoring and immunosuppressive treatment do not form part of this work.

The operation itself is not difficult but must be performed carefully in order to reduce the incidence of technical complications, which are probably higher than most transplant surgeons would like to admit. There is a choice of two possible donors: one a cadaver donor, the other a living volunteer.

Donor operation

Cadaver donor

Most kidneys are removed from patients who have died from head injury or cerebrovascular catastrophe in whom complete and irreversible death of the brain stem has been demonstrated according to accepted criteria[1] [2].

Increasingly common now is removal of multiple organs from the same donor, often the wish of the relatives. We have on a number of occasions removed both kidneys, liver, pancreas and heart as well as the corneas from the same donor, and all have functioned satisfactorily when transplanted into their respective recipients. Careful and time-consuming dissection is required. A bilateral subcostal incision is made and if the heart is to be removed, a vertical extension includes division of the sternum in the midline.

A category of donor that is uncommon now is the patient who is brought in dead, usually from a road traffic accident, stroke, or myocardial infarct. In such cases rapid removal of kidneys within one hour of cardiac arrest is essential; damage may be minimised by inserting a triple lumen double-balloon catheter into a femoral artery, passing it into the aorta and inflating the lowermost balloon. The catheter is pulled back so that the distended balloon is sited at the aortic bifurcation. The upper balloon is then inflated and it should lie at the level of the diaphragm. Through the intervening portion of the catheter between the two balloons cold preservation fluid is infused, which will cool the organs supplied by the abdominal aorta. While this cold infusion is in progress the kidneys are removed as quickly as possible and plunged into ice-cold saline.

Preservation technique

Once removed, whether from a living or dead donor, the cold preservation technique is the same. The kidney lies in a bowl of normal saline at 4°C and the renal artery is cannulated by hand. The cannula is attached to tubing connected to a bag containing hypertonic citrate solution at 4°C on a dripstand approximately one metre above the kidney. Perfusion through the renal artery continues until the surface of the kidney blanches and the effluent from the renal vein contains no macroscopic blood. 200–300 ml of perfusion fluid may be needed. The kidney is then double-wrapped in sterile bags and surrounded by ice and can be kept with confidence for 24 hours. There may be a little damage in the kidney preserved between 24 to 48 hours if the period of warm ischaemia is short and the anastomoses in the recipient done rapidly, say within 20 minutes for the artery and vein. Longer periods of preservation by this simple method should be avoided, because damage will probably be severe.

Living donor

To remove a kidney from a healthy individual should not be undertaken lightly. We require that the donor is a blood relative, who has at least one haplotype of antigens in common with the recipient, for example parent to child. There must be no evidence of disease in the cardiovascular system or renal tract, and no demonstrable antibodies in the recipient against donor lymphocytes. We spend time with the donor and the family to determine that the giving of the kidney is a positive desire of the would-be donor and that he is not being subjected to pressure within the family. The pain of the operation and the definite risks involved are not minimised, nor the possibility that the graft may fail.

After careful medical examination an arteriogram is performed with free flush of contrast in the aorta to show the anatomy of the renal arteries. Multiple arteries are common and their presence compromises the chances of success. Especially important is a lower polar vessel which usually is a major contributor to the blood supply of the renal pelvis and the ureter of the transplanted kidney. A kidney with a single artery is best and if there are multiple arteries on both sides, the donor may be unsuitable because a patch of aorta containing the orifices of both renal arteries cannot be taken from a living donor.

Under general anaesthesia, with the patient in the lateral position, an intravenous infusion of Mannitol is started. The kidney is approached in the extraperitoneal plane through the bed of the twelfth rib, the distal portion of which is excised. If both kidneys have normal anatomy the left one is preferable because the renal vein is longer. After ligation and division of the renal vessels and ureter, the kidney is plunged into ice-cold saline and perfused with cold hypertonic citrate solution as for a kidney taken from a cadaver donor.

Recipient operation

In adults the kidney is placed in the iliac fossa in the extraperitoneal plane. In small children it may be necessary to use the peritoneal cavity. An arterial inflow is established from the systemic arterial system and venous drainage into the inferior vena caval system. Although a right or left kidney may be grafted to either side, the anatomy of the renal vessels and ureter make certain procedures preferable.

To avoid lymphatic leakage postoperatively, perivascular dissection is limited to provide sufficient mobility of the vessels for clamping and anastomosis. Any lymphatics that have to be divided are ligated with fine catgut. If a patch of aorta has been included, which is usually the case from a cadaver donor, the kidney is most conveniently transplanted to the homolateral side, the anastomoses being made end-to-side to the external iliac vessels.

From a live donor, transplantation to the contralateral side may be preferred, anastomosing the renal artery end-to-end to the proximal divided end of the internal iliac artery, the distal end being ligated. It is important to exclude severe atherosclerosis of the internal iliac artery, which may make arterial inflow to the kidney unsatisfactory. Venous drainage is to the external iliac vein with an end-to-side anastomosis.

For children, especially when a large kidney is transplanted into a small child, an intraperitoneal abdominal approach is used and the renal vessels are anastomosed end-to-side to the common iliac vessels or the aorta and vena cava. In all cases the ureter is implanted into the bladder near the dome with a submucous tunnel of approximately 2 cm in length. If the kidney has suffered from warm ischaemia, as have many transplants from cadaver donors, the ureter is splinted with a No. 6 Tizzard catheter brought out through the dome of the bladder and a stab incision in the skin. The splint being left in place for 5 days before removal, a retrograde injection of contrast is given, and an xray is taken to show that the graft drainage is satisfactory. The urinary catheter is removed between the 7th and 10th day.

From a live donor splintage of the ureter is usually not necessary. A small biopsy is taken from the lower pole of the kidney to provide the pathologist with a specimen for a baseline reference which may be used for comparison with future biopsies. In donation from a cadaver, the renal capsule is incised longitudinally to permit renal swelling that may result if there is an episode of acute rejection. The wound is drained with a Silastic tube drain 1 cm in diameter brought out through the upper extremity of the wound incision.

The donor and recipient operations usually take between one and two hours each, unless the donor has been brought in dead, in which case kidney removal is as rapid as possible.

The objective of the surgeon should be to ensure the shortest time when the kidney is warm and unperfused both in the donor and the recipient. Dissection is deliberate and gentle so as not to damage the delicate organs and their blood vessels.

Special hazards

1   It is especially important to leave the periureteric connective tissue intact, because the blood supply to the lower end of the ureter coming from the renal artery may be precarious.

2   The placement of the anastomosis on the iliac vessels should be considered not only from the point of view of the ease with which the

surgeon can perform the anastomoses, but also how the vessels and the kidney will lie when the wound is closed. Thus the renal artery and vein should be unhampered, without kinking or twisting. If the renal vein is too long, closure of the wound may compress the renal substance against the vein and cause venous obstruction. If the renal vein is too short, it may be very difficult to join it to the iliac vein; this applies especially on the right side where the renal vein is only 2 cm in length.

3   In removing the donor kidney it is important not to pull the kidney upwards with any force to facilitate dissection. Traction can lead to rupture of the intima, which then curls up inside the renal artery leading to primary or early failure of arterial inflow to the kidney, often misinterpreted as 'hyperacute rejection' by inexperienced surgeons.

4   Any handling of the vascular intima of the donor or recipient vessels should be reduced to a minimum, and special atraumatic forceps should be used if possible. A strabismus hook is often preferable to forceps, to hold open the lumen of the vessels being anastomosed.

5   The details of the operation should be always carefully recorded. It is helpful to do this with a line diagram so that if re-exploration of the kidney is needed at a later date, the arrangement of the anatomy can be anticipated. After the kidney has been in place for some weeks, there is considerable fibrotic reaction around the organ even without significant rejection or infection. This can make re-exploration hazardous and there may be danger of the kidney prolapsing out of the wound and tearing the anastomoses apart, especially if relaxation of the abdominal wall muscles has been inadequate.

The techniques illustrated here are not claimed to be comprehensive. Most surgical operations can be performed in a variety of ways. I have portrayed the typical procedure in our unit. Illustrations have attempted to show the operation as seen by the surgeon, with examples of some common anatomical anomalies.

Acknowledgements

My thanks to colleagues who have helped with the photographs in the operating theatre and to the Department of Medical Illustration and Photography, Addenbrooke's Hospital, in preparing the transparencies.

I am also grateful to Mr Neville Jamieson and Mr Robert Greatorex for their constructive suggestions.

Donor operation

1 Arteriogram of potential live donor showing the coeliac, renal and lumbar vessels as well as the aorta. On the left side there is one renal artery, on the right one main renal artery and an artery to the lower pole probably supplying the renal pelvis and upper ureter. The left kidney was therefore used.

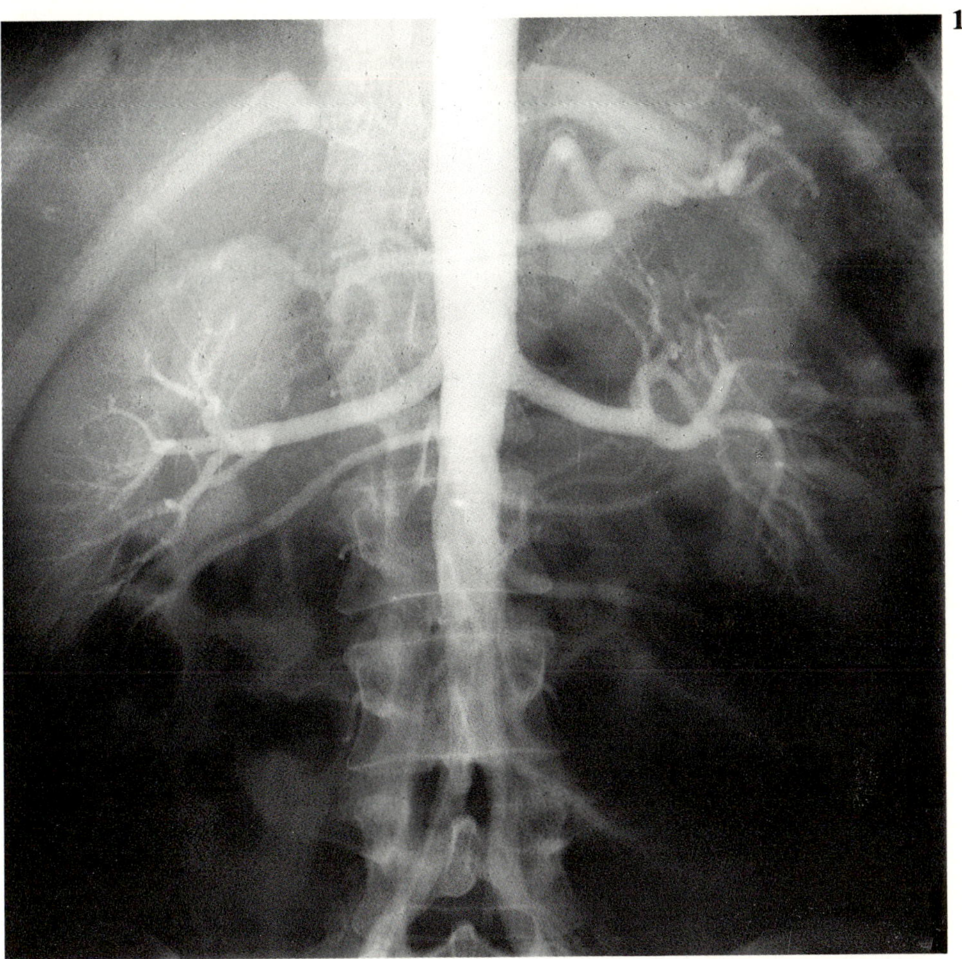

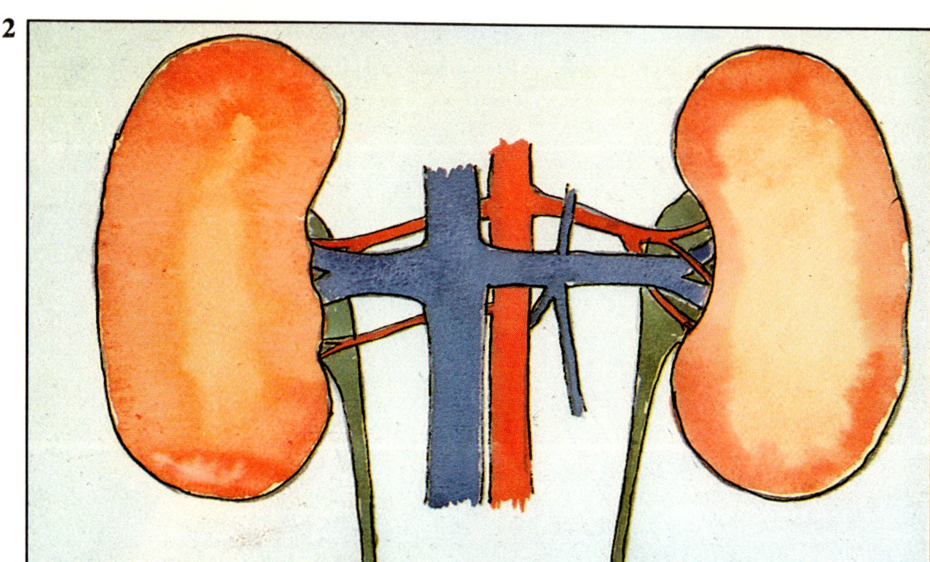

2   The anatomy of the kidneys, ureters and their blood vessels shown in 1. On the left there is one artery, one vein and one ureter. The renal vein is long and three moderate-sized branches converge to join it. They are above the adrenal, below and medial a large lumbar vein, and below and lateral the left gonadal vein. These vessels require ligation and division in the removal of the kidney.

Depicted in this diagram are two right renal arteries, the upper main artery and the lower extra vessel which supplies the renal pelvis and upper ureter.

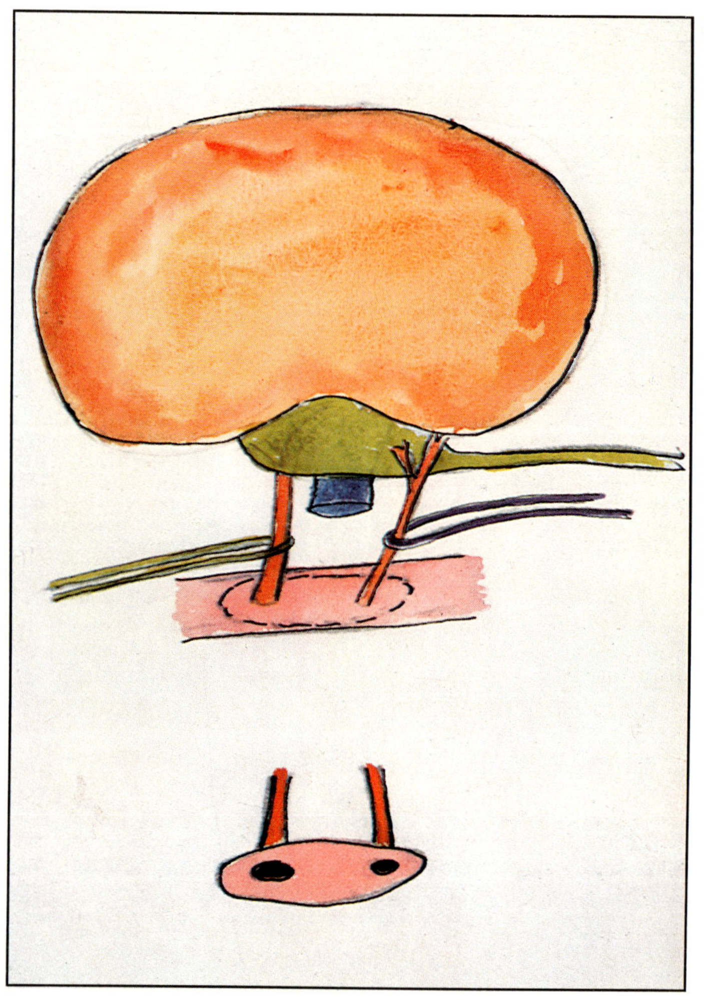

3   If the anatomy shown in 2 is encountered in a cadaver donor, the two renal vessels are removed on one Carrel patch.

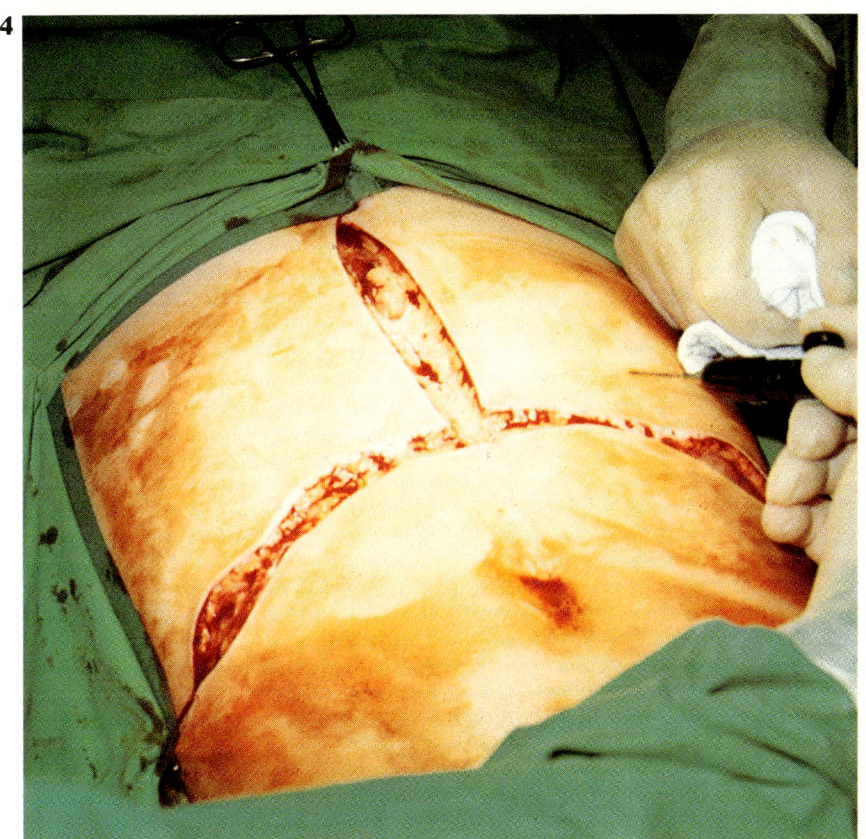

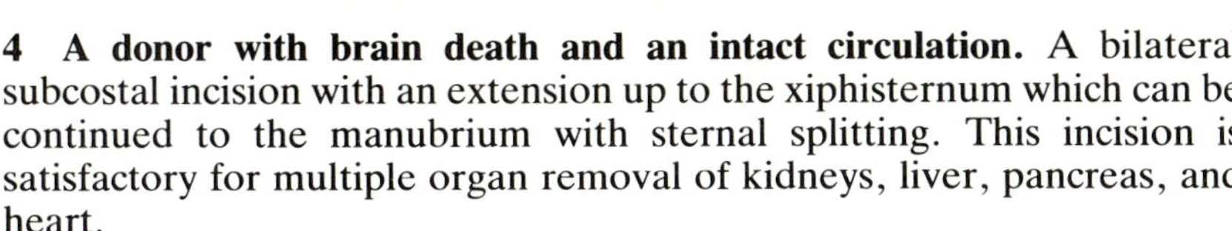

4 A donor with brain death and an intact circulation. A bilateral subcostal incision with an extension up to the xiphisternum which can be continued to the manubrium with sternal splitting. This incision is satisfactory for multiple organ removal of kidneys, liver, pancreas, and heart.

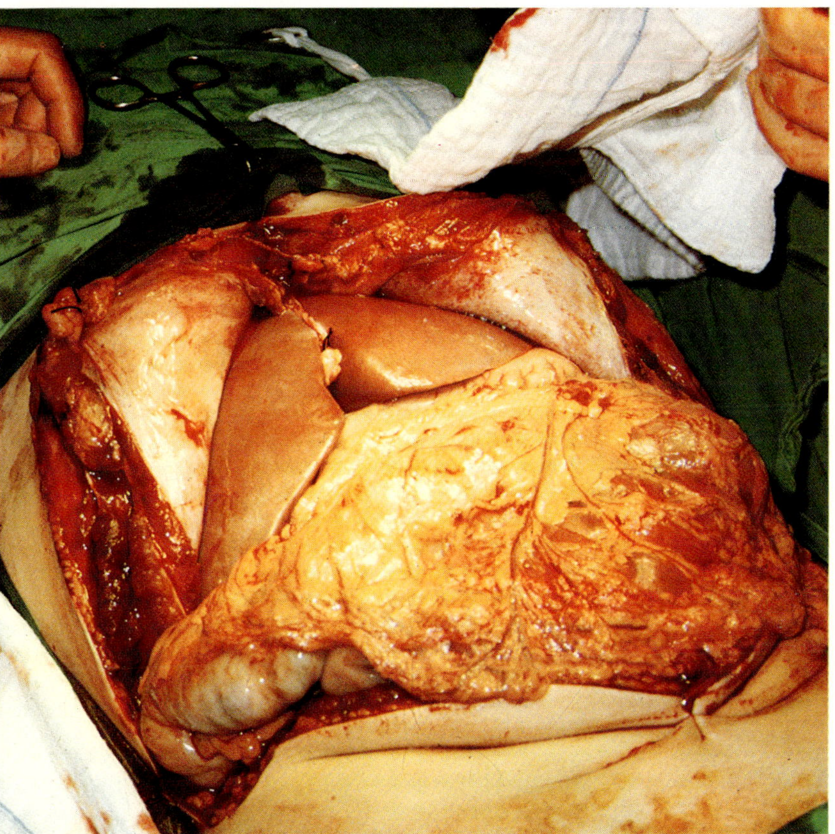

5 The incision has been made through the abdominal wall, the upper flaps have been sutured to the skin below the nipples, and the lower flap to the skin above the pubis. This provides excellent access for the upper abdominal organs.

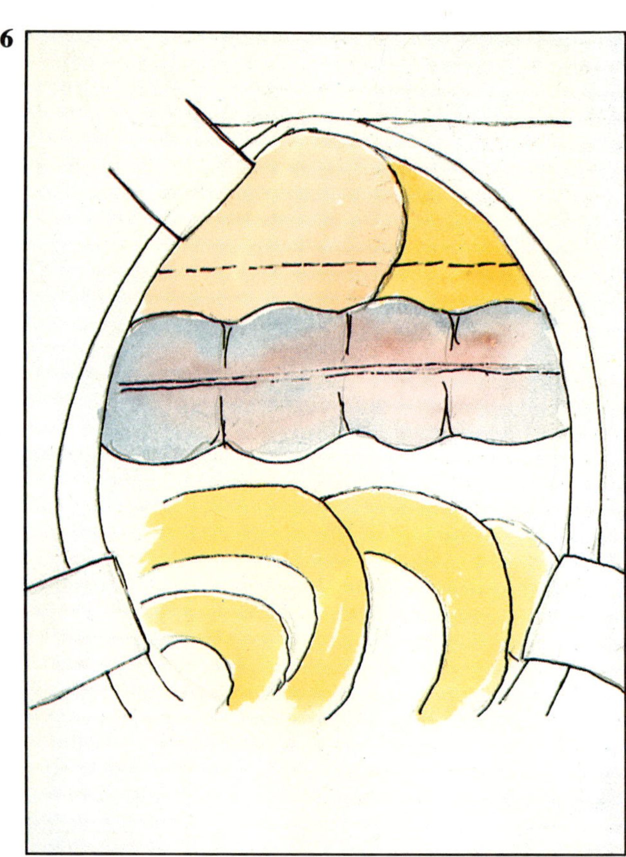

6 Diagram to show incision (viewed from the right) in parietal peritoneum posteriorly, lateral to the descending colon which is mobilised and brought medially to allow exposure of the left kidney.

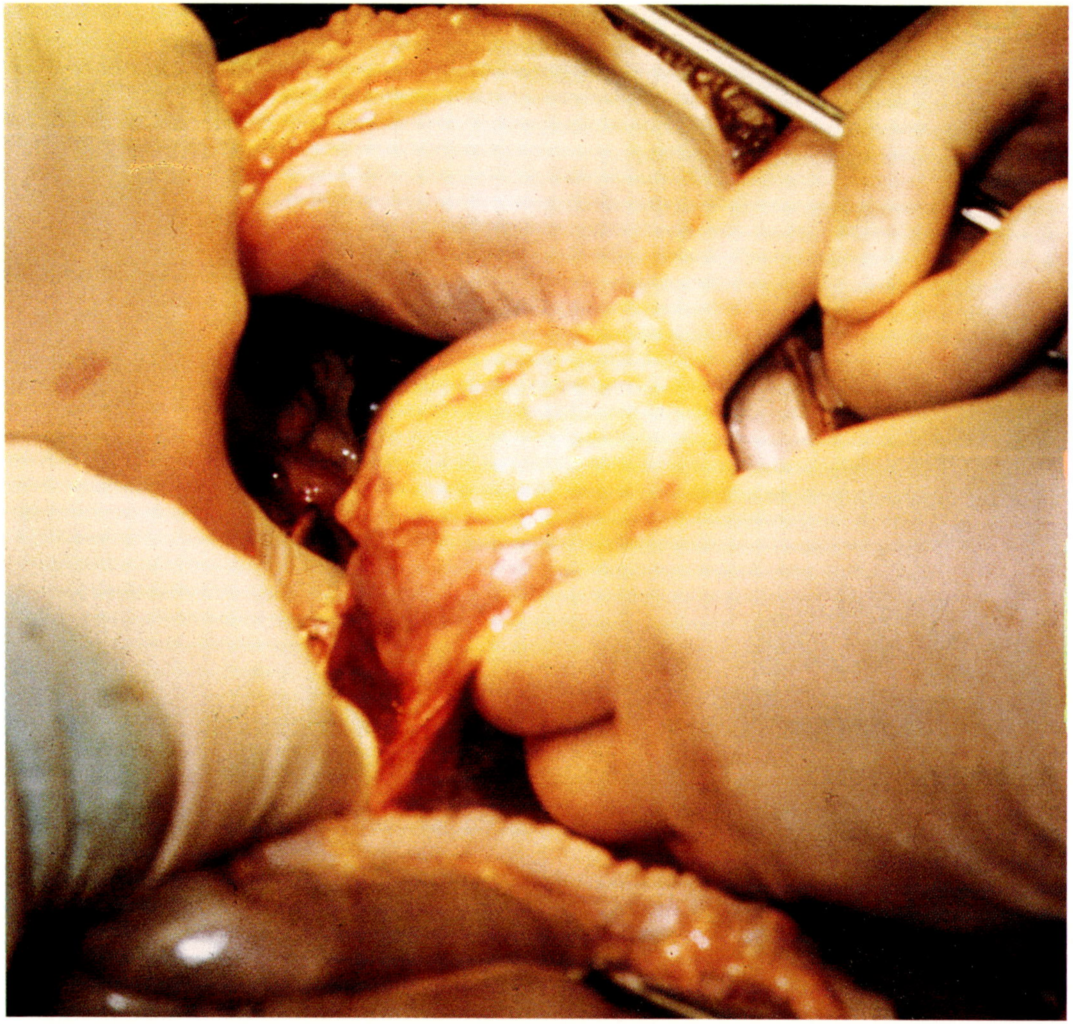

7 The left kidney is mobilised. Peri-renal tissue is divided.

8 The left kidney viewed from the left. The renal vein can be seen with a red sling around it. There is a yellow sling around the renal artery which cannot be well visualised, and there are ties in position around the gonadal and adrenal veins.

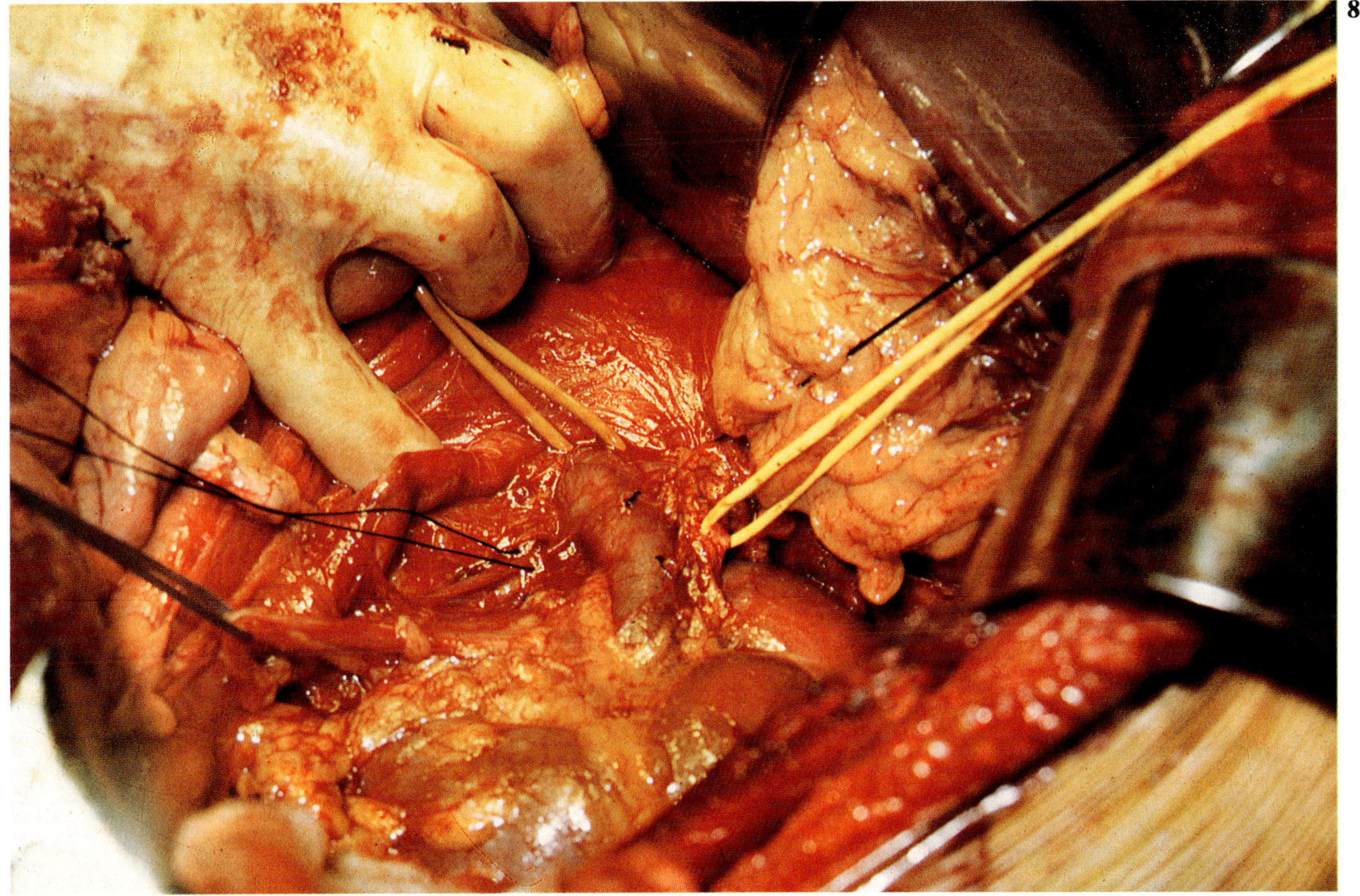

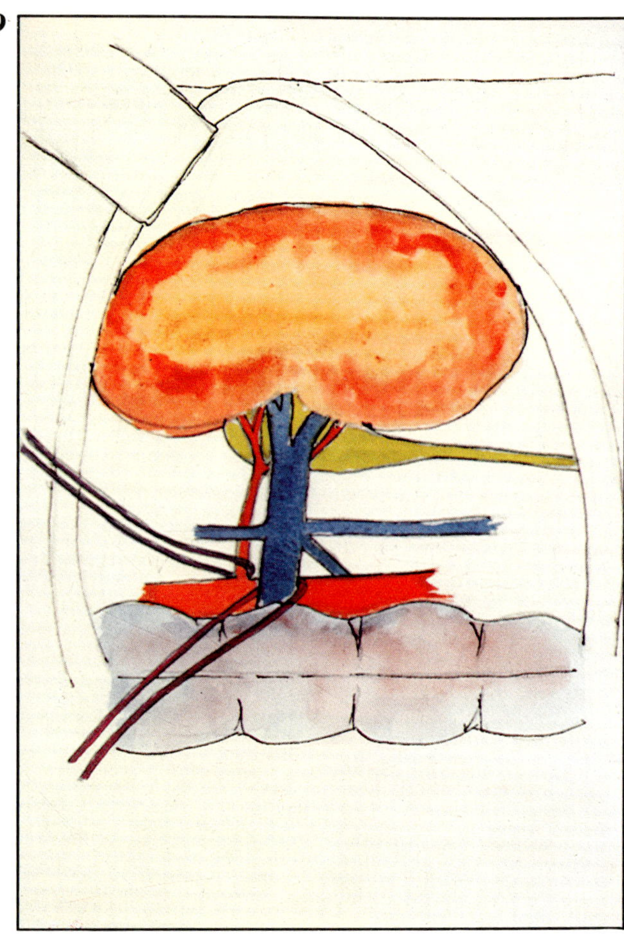

9   **Diagram of soft-rubber slings being passed around the left renal vein medial to the three branches** and around the renal artery close to the aorta. Left kidney viewed from the right.

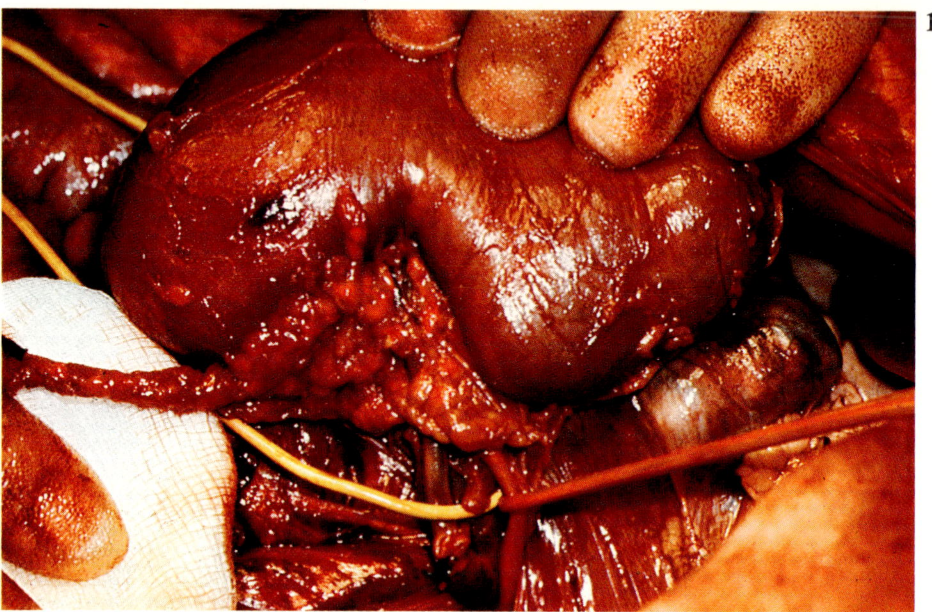

10   **The left kidney has been lifted up and is viewed from behind.** There is a red sling around the renal artery and a yellow one around the renal vein. The ureter can be seen to the left on top of a white swab.

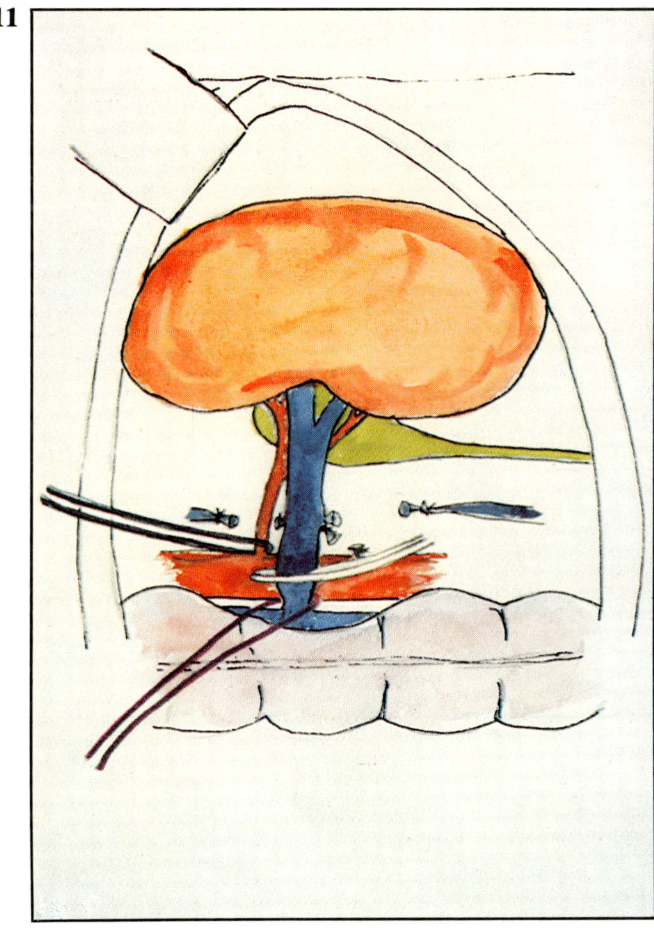

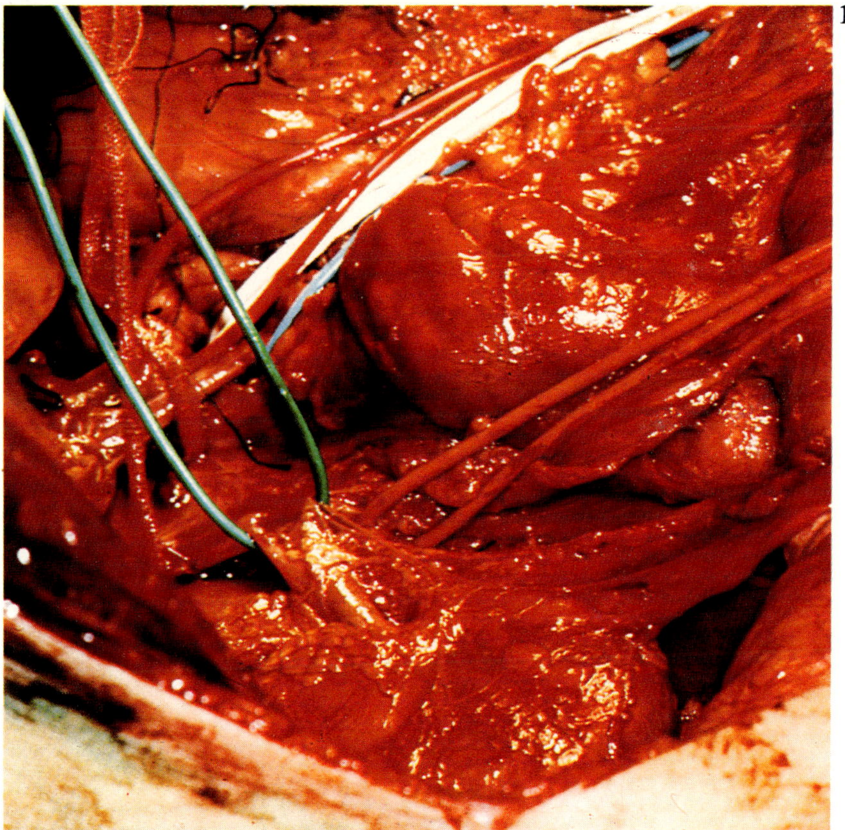

12   A green sling has been passed around the right renal vein and a red sling around the renal artery. The ureter can be seen to the right. Slings can also be seen around the structures in the free edge of the lesser omentum. These are concerned with removal of the liver and are not part of the donor kidney operation.

11   Diagram of the left kidney fully mobilised. The left renal vein is about to be divided with scissors, close to the inferior vena cava. If bleeding is anticipated, the renal vein can be clamped at the cava with a vascular clamp and a soft bulldog clip applied to the renal vein near the hilum. A Carrel patch of aorta is normally taken with the renal artery even if there is only one main renal artery. If there is a long distance between two renal arteries, two Carrel patches may be necessary. If there are more than two independent main renal arteries, the chances of a vascular complication are increased.

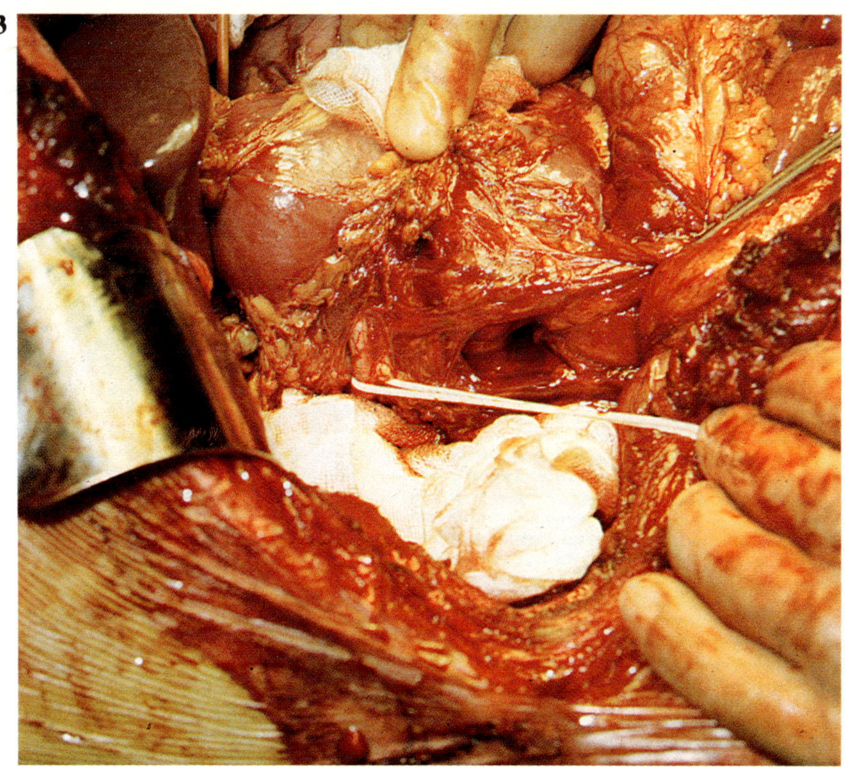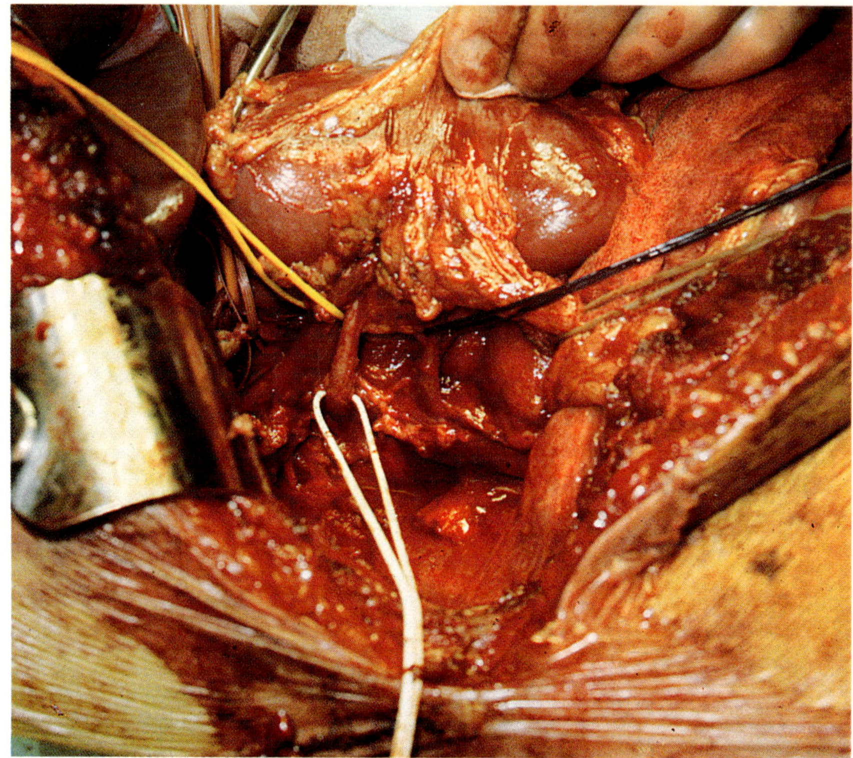

13 The right kidney viewed from the right. The organ has been lifted forward. There are slings around the ureter (brown) and the renal artery (white).

14 Further dissection of the right kidney with the main renal vein above with a yellow sling and an additional lower renal vein with a blue sling. Slings around the portal vein and hepatic artery can be seen above the kidney between it and the liver.

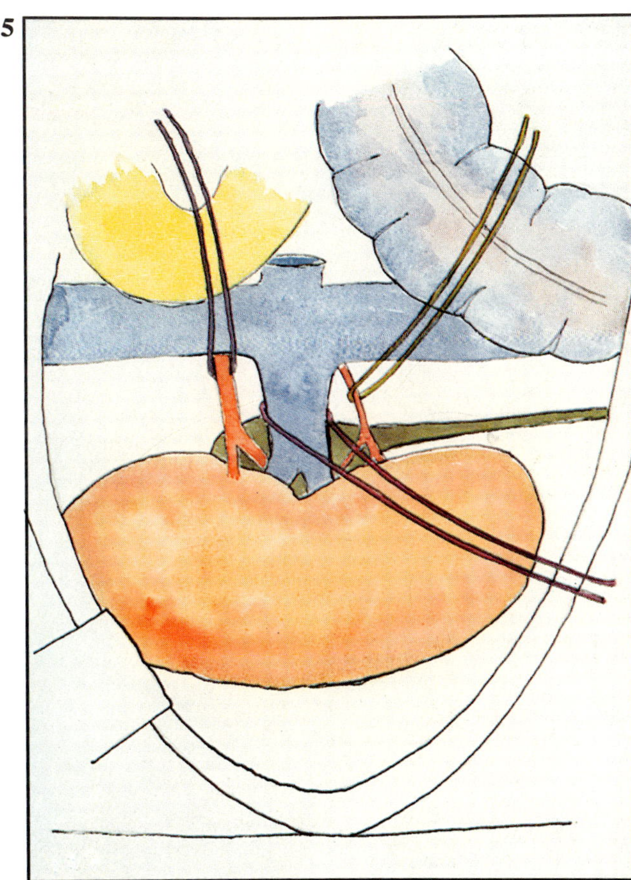

15   **Diagram of mobilisation of the right kidney with a purple sling around the renal vein,** the main renal artery above and the polar vessel supplying the renal pelvis and upper ureter below. The duodenum and hepatic flexure of the colon have been mobilised medially.

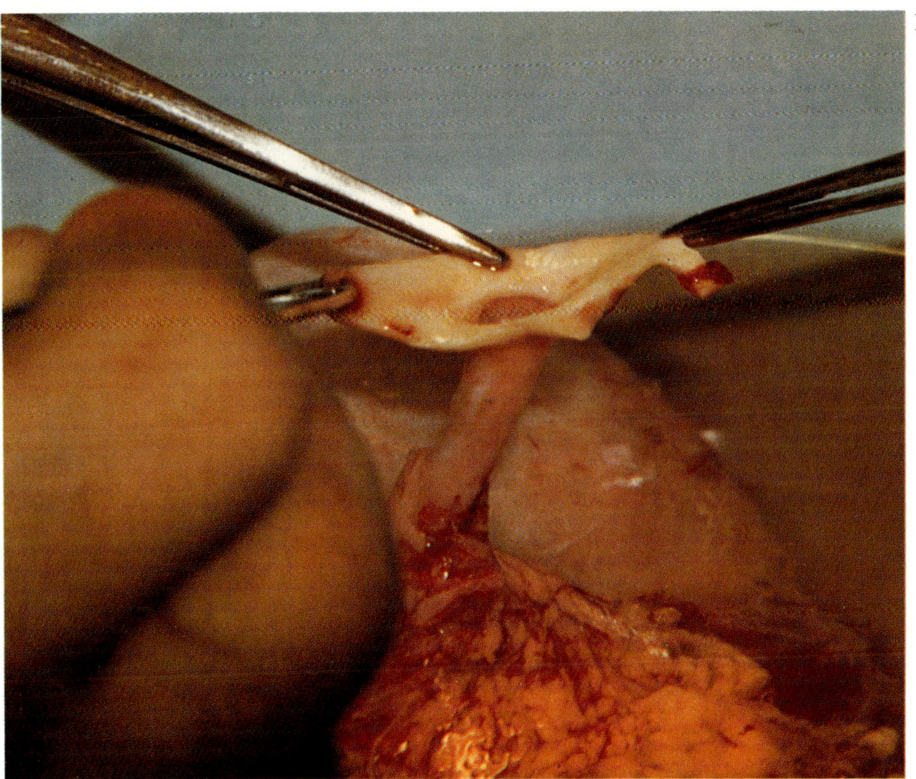

16   **The kidney having been removed, is plunged into a plastic dish filled with ice-cold saline.** The Carrel patch of aorta containing the renal artery is inspected and the patch can be trimmed at this stage to provide just enough rim of aorta to take the anastomotic stitches.

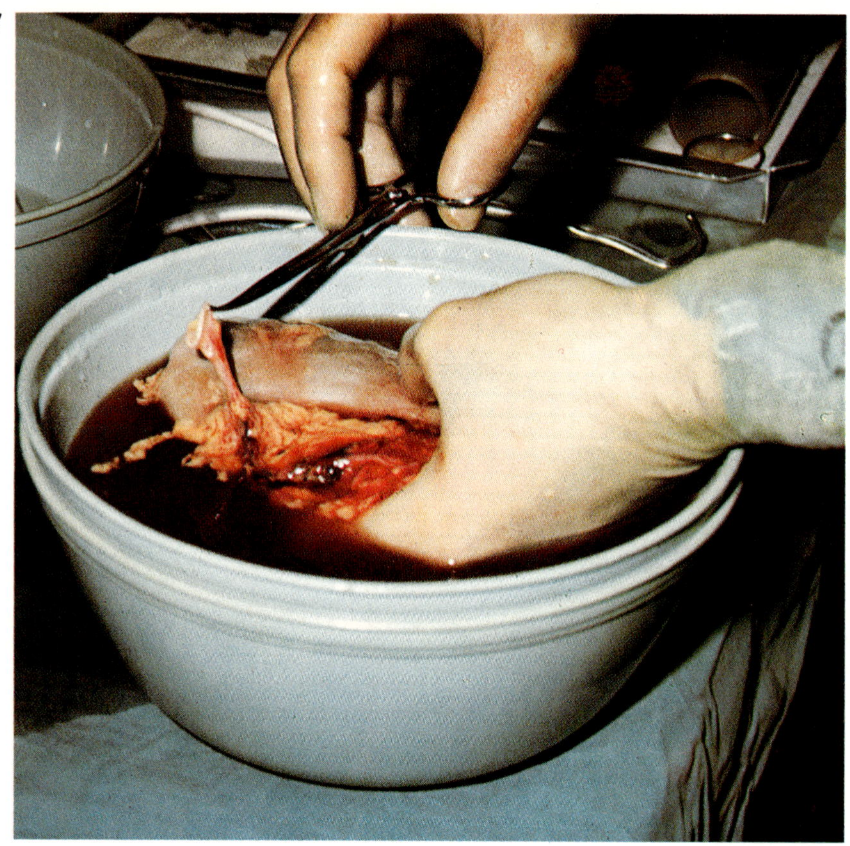

17 The Carrel patch is now held in a Mosquito forceps ready for cannulation and perfusion of the kidney.

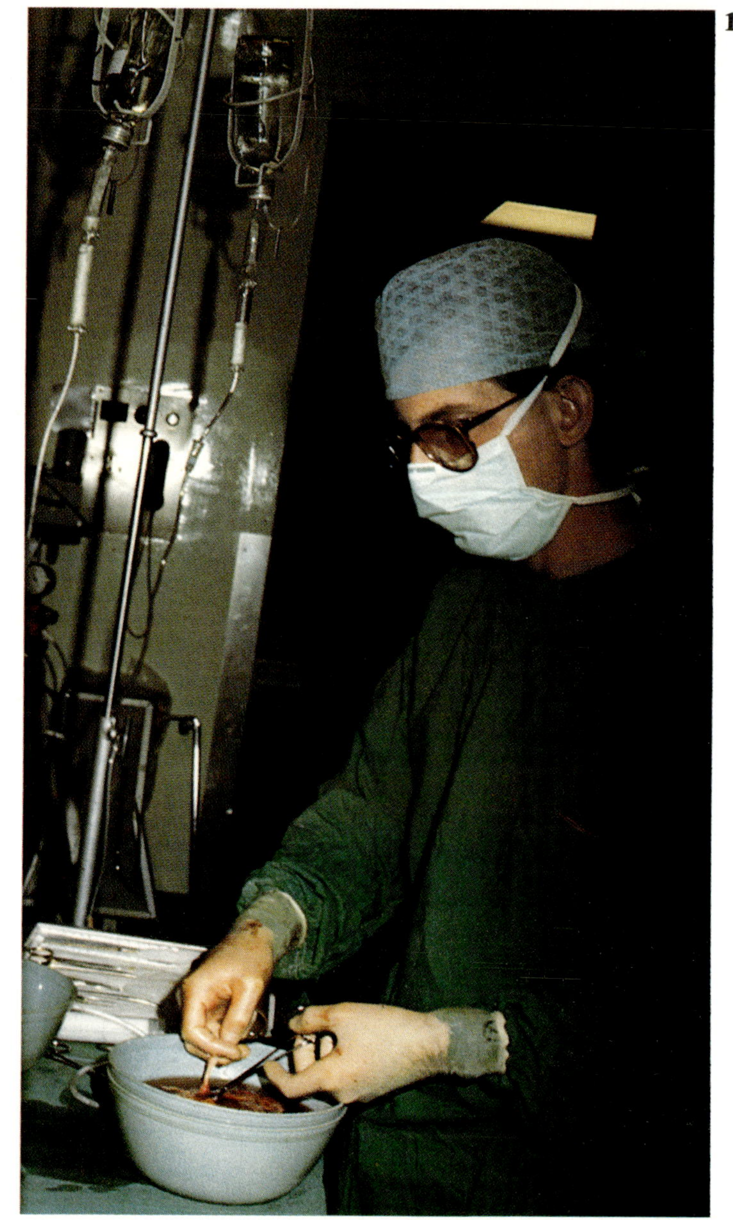

18 Shows the cool preserving fluid (hypertonic citrate) at 4°C approximately one metre above the kidney, being infused into the renal artery. A plastic cannula is held gently between the fingers and thumb in the lumen of the renal artery. Effluent from the renal vein has coloured the saline dark red.

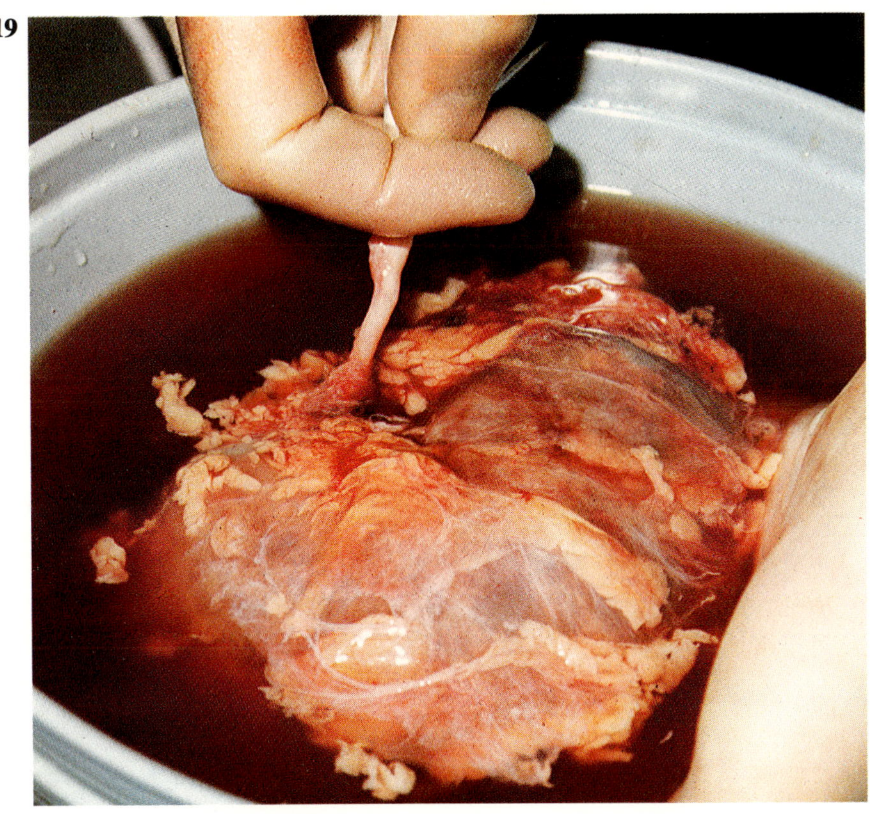

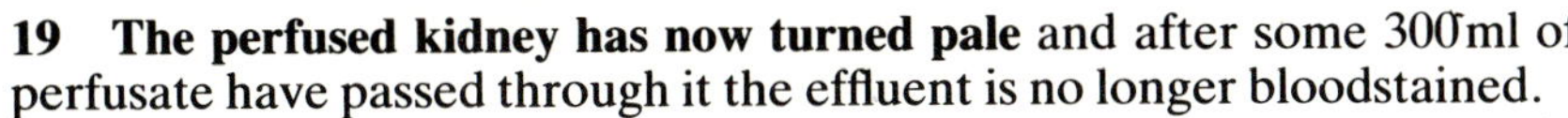

19 The perfused kidney has now turned pale and after some 300 ml of perfusate have passed through it the effluent is no longer bloodstained.

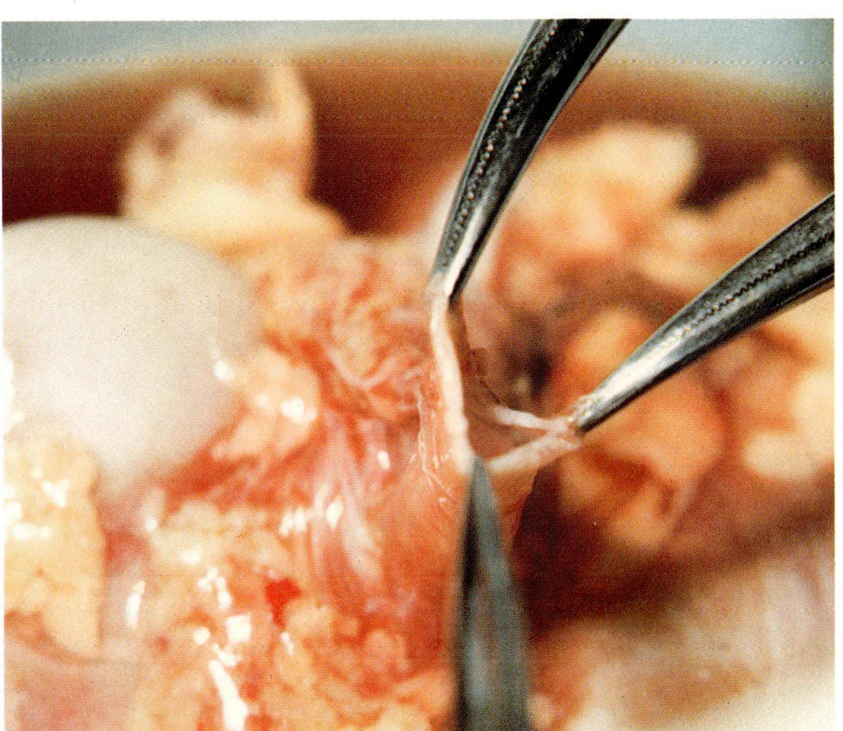

20 The renal vein is inspected and its anatomy scrutinised.

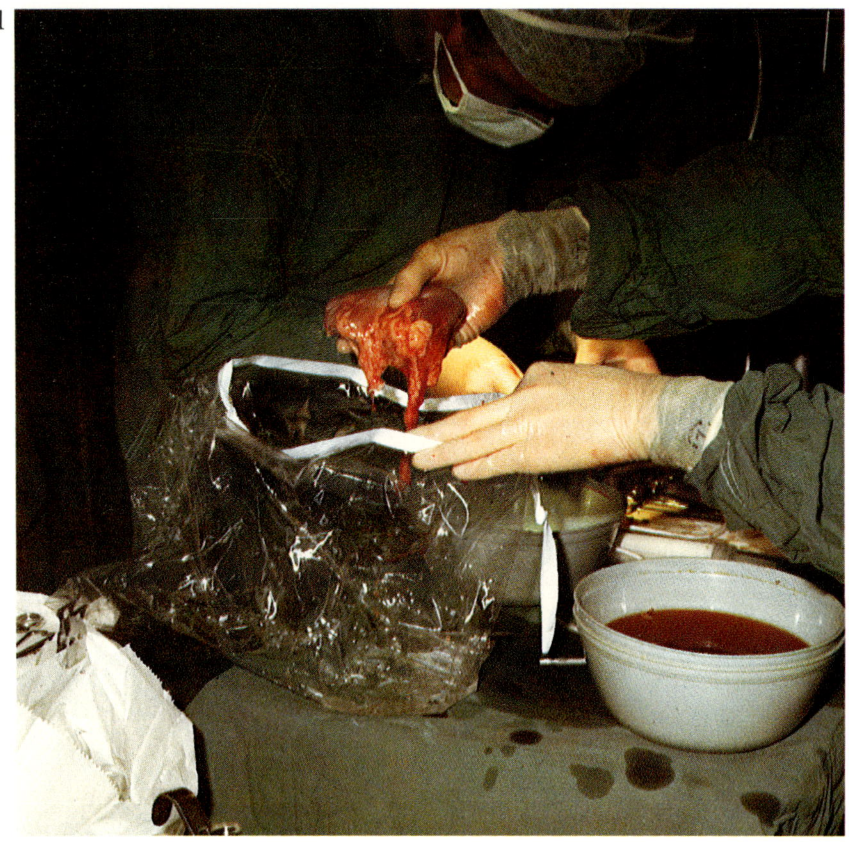

21 **The kidney is now placed in a sterile plastic bag containing ice-cold saline.**

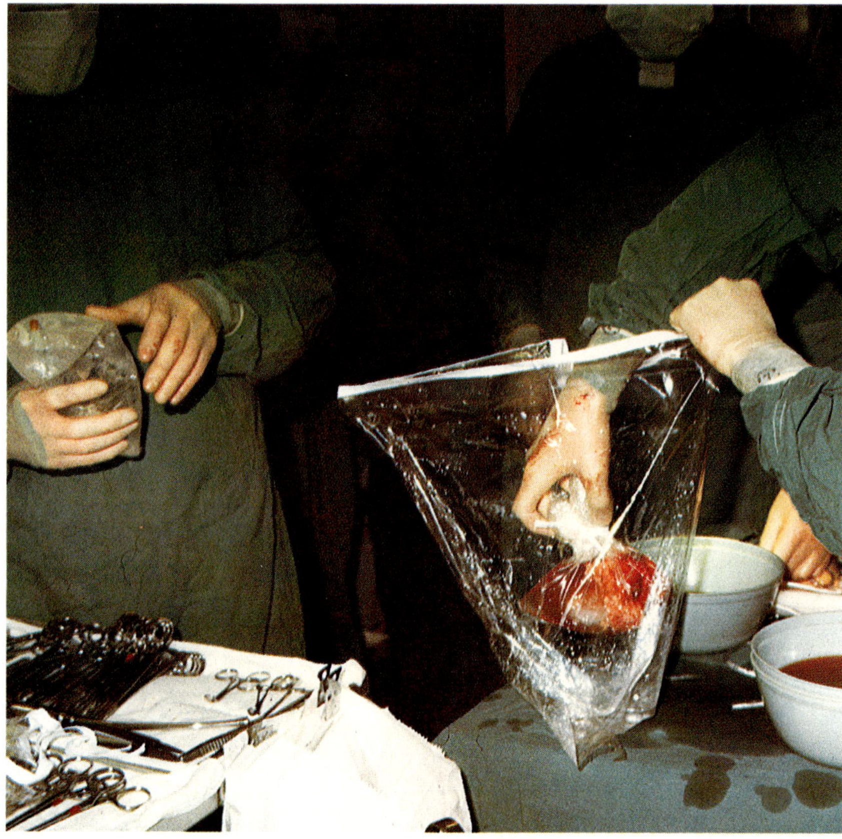

22 **The bag is closed by tying a tape around its neck and expelling all air and is inserted into another similar bag which is treated likewise.** The outside of the second bag will not remain sterile, because it will be in contact with ordinary ice in the ice box.

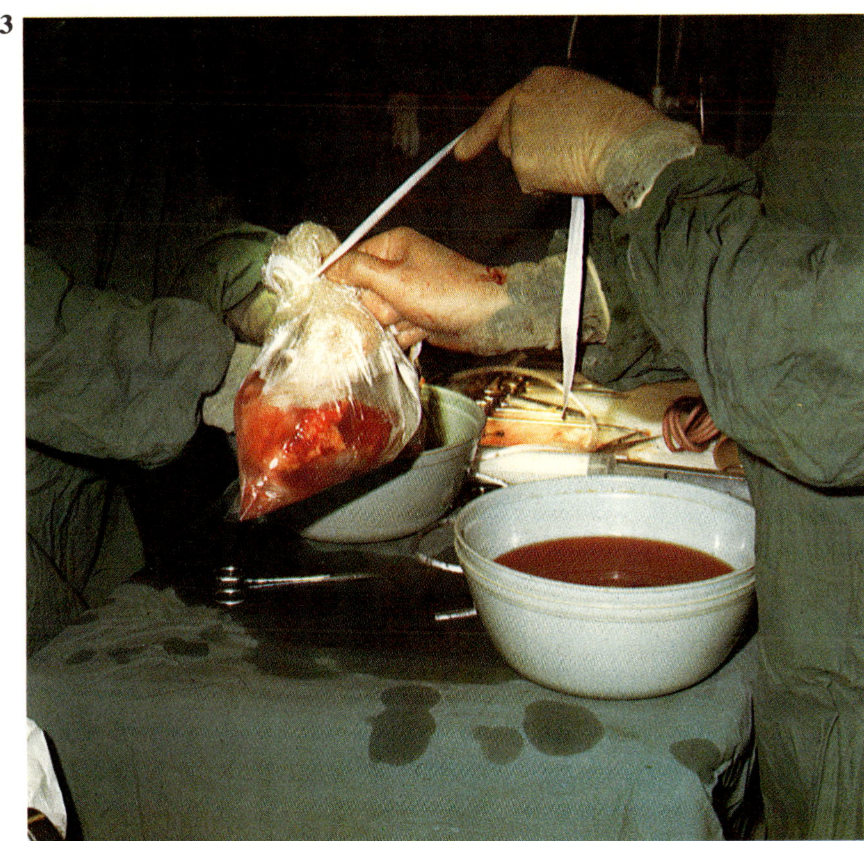

23 The neck of the second bag is closed with a tight tape wound around it and tied.

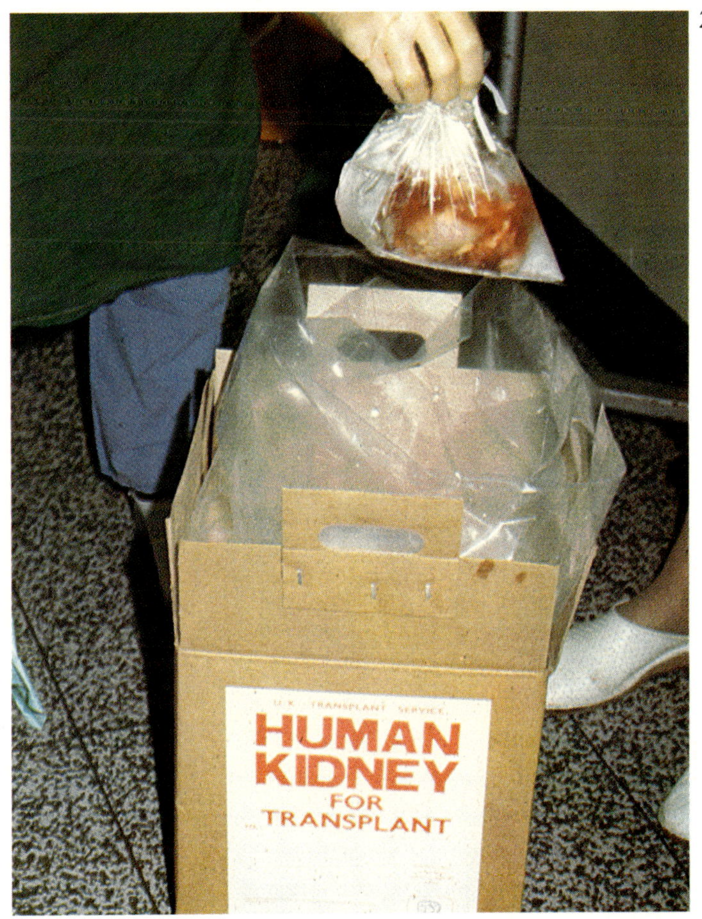

24 The kidney within its two bags is now inserted into the polystyrene box containing ice below, and ice is loosely packed around and on top of the kidney.

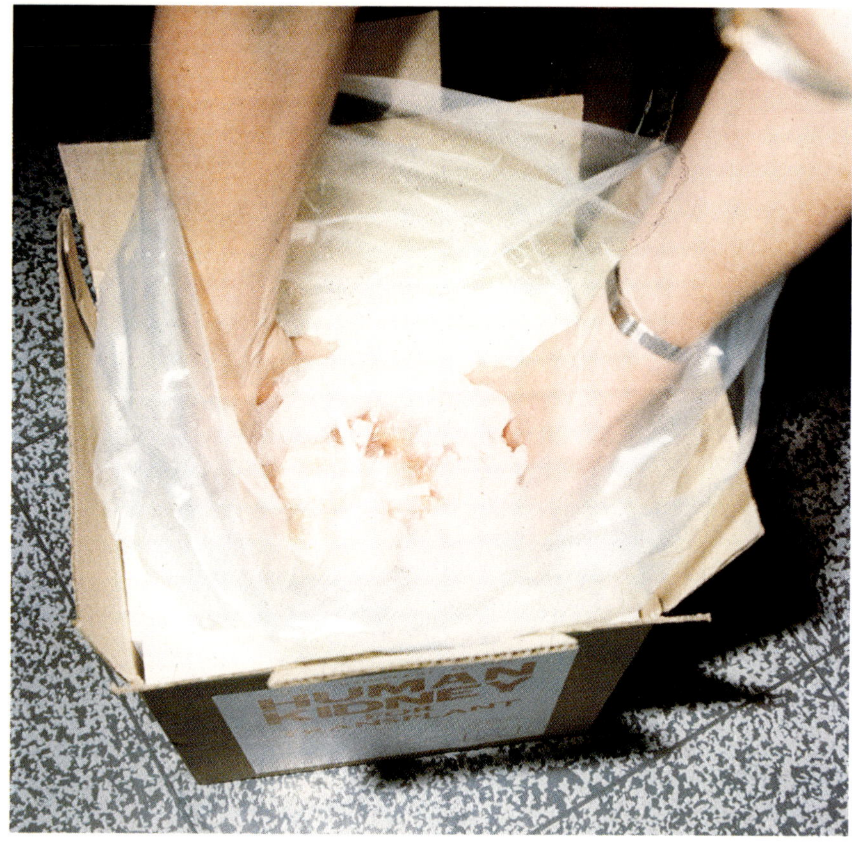

25 The outer bag is now surrounded by ice and the box is ready for closing. The kidney will keep in good condition for up to 48 hours provided the condition of the donor when the kidney was removed was satisfactory, and there was not a significant period when the kidney was warm and ischaemic before the perfusion of cold fluid started.

Live donor operation

Removal of the left kidney

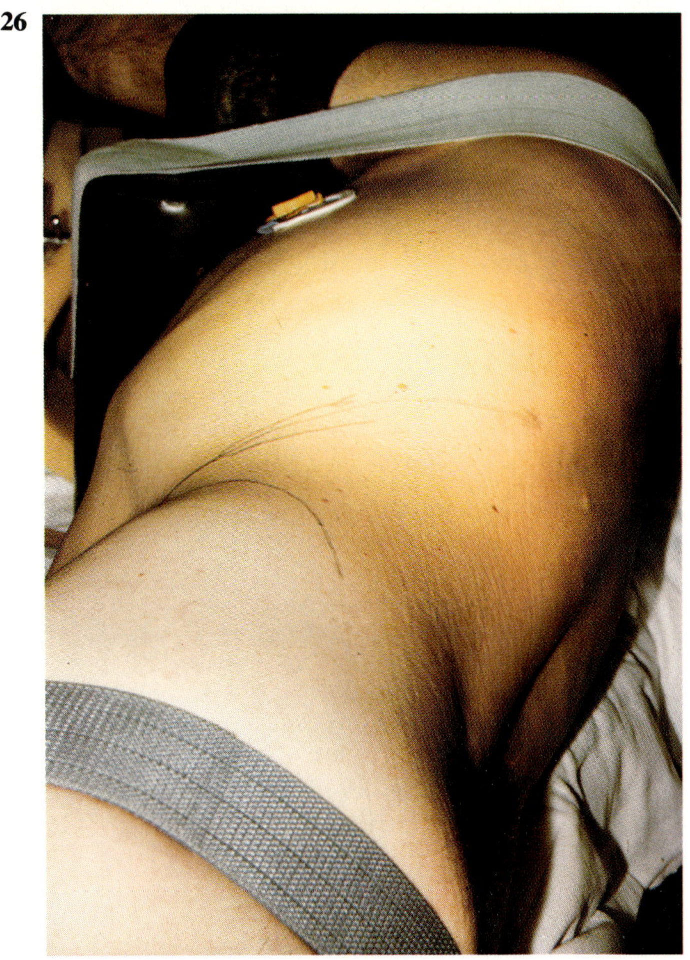

26   The patient is in the left lateral position viewed from behind. The left twelfth rib has been outlined as has the iliac crest.

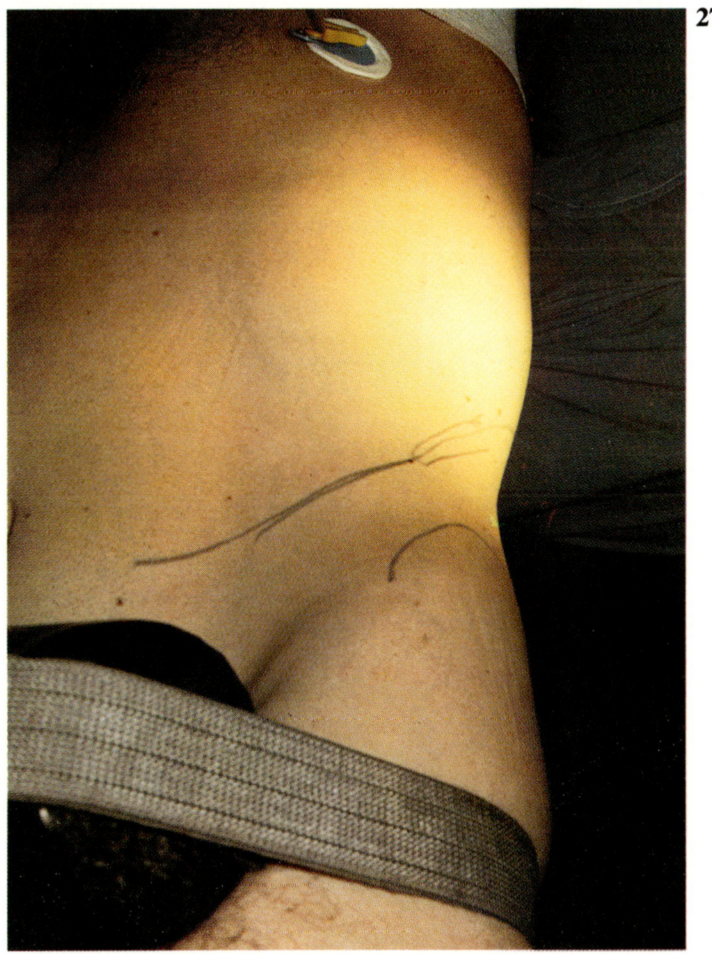

27   Shows continuation of the line of the incision from the tip of the twelfth rib down towards the umbilicus viewed from the front.

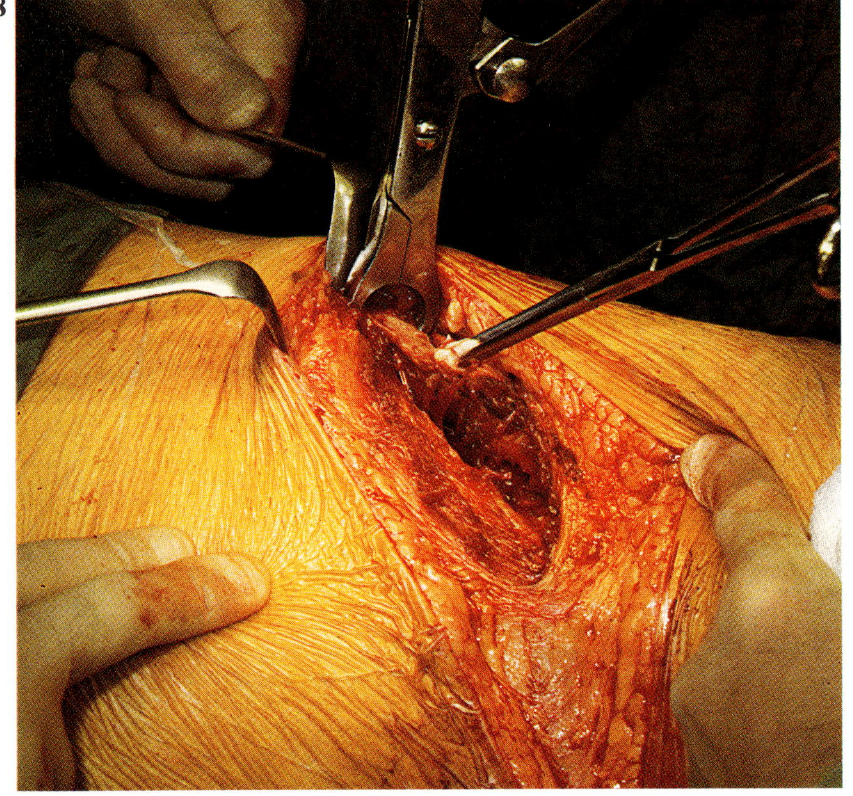

28   The incision has been made. The periosteum has been stripped from the distal portion of the twelfth rib and the rib shears are in position. The tip of the rib is held with Kocher's forceps.

29   The shears have been closed and the distal portion of the rib is being removed.

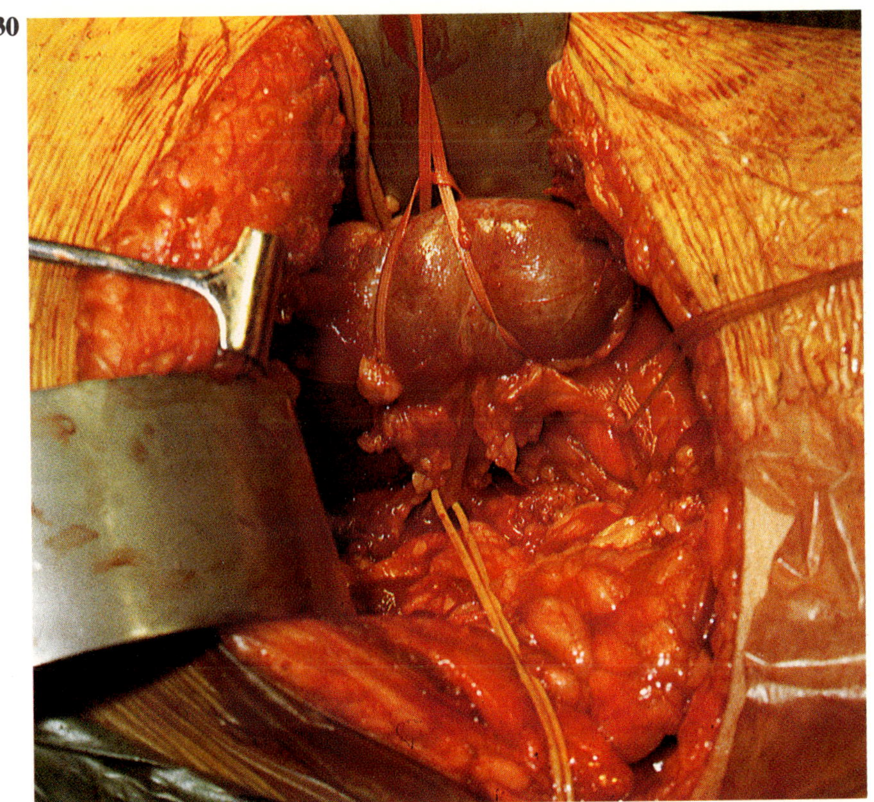

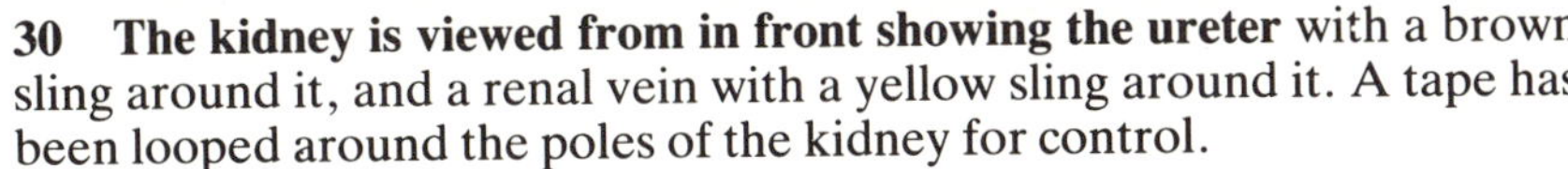

30 **The kidney is viewed from in front showing the ureter** with a brown sling around it, and a renal vein with a yellow sling around it. A tape has been looped around the poles of the kidney for control.

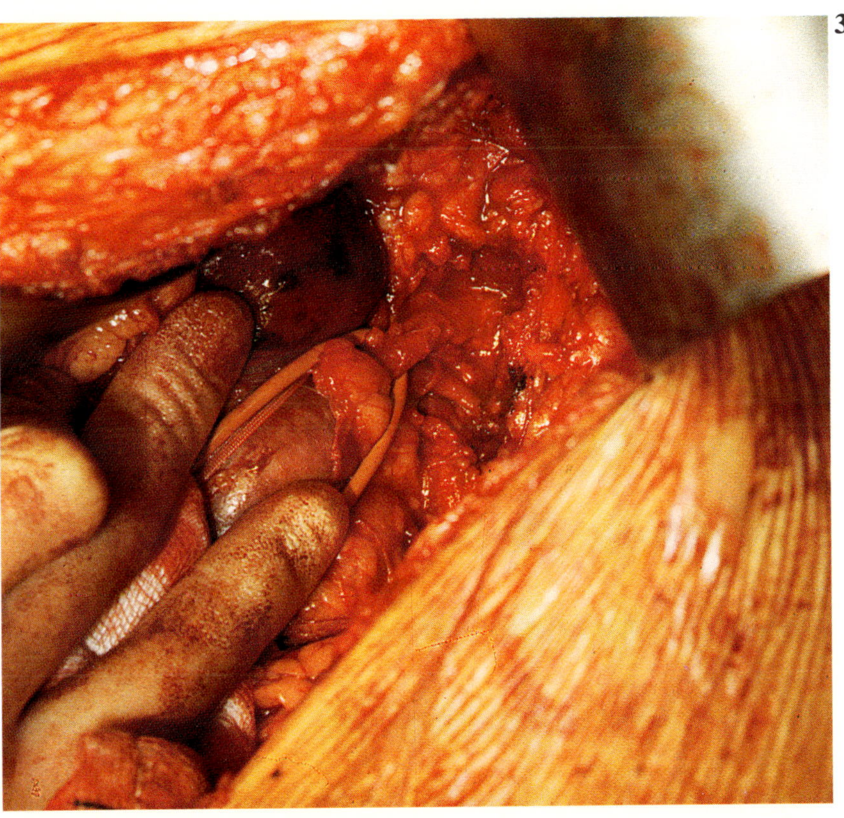

31 **Shows the commencement of the dissection of the renal artery from behind.** The artery is controlled with a red sling.

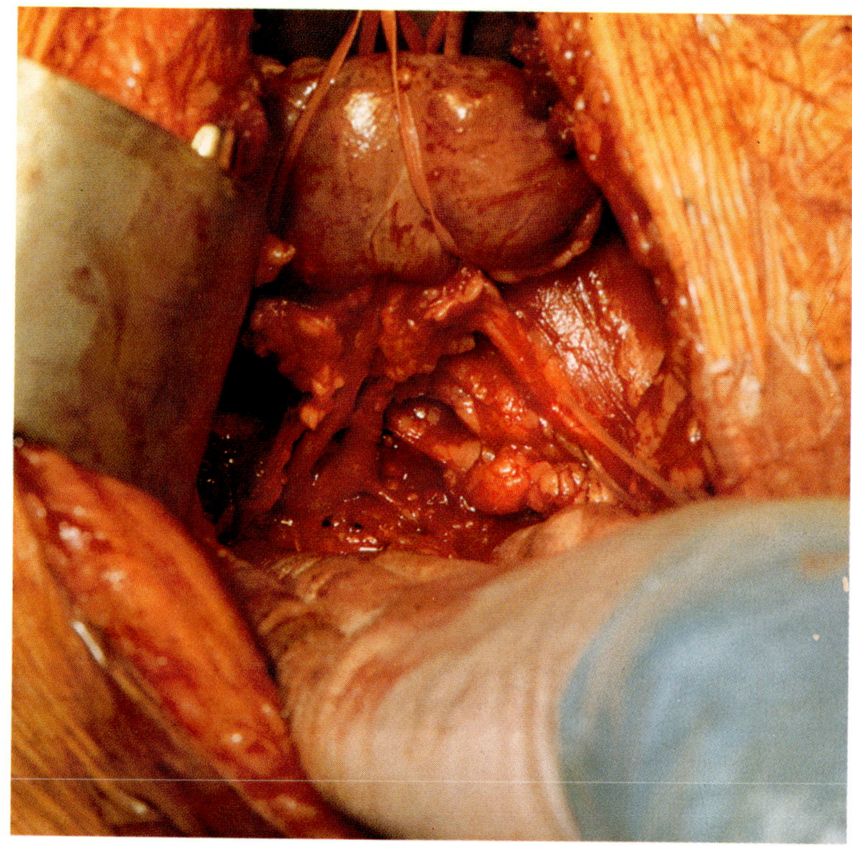

32   **The venous anatomy has now been demonstrated and is abnormal.**
There are two renal veins, the gonadal enters the lower renal vein and
the adrenal the upper. The two veins join into a common trunk in front
of the aorta. The common renal vein will be ligated and divided
overlying the right margin of the aorta close to the vena cava.

Recipient operation

Adult

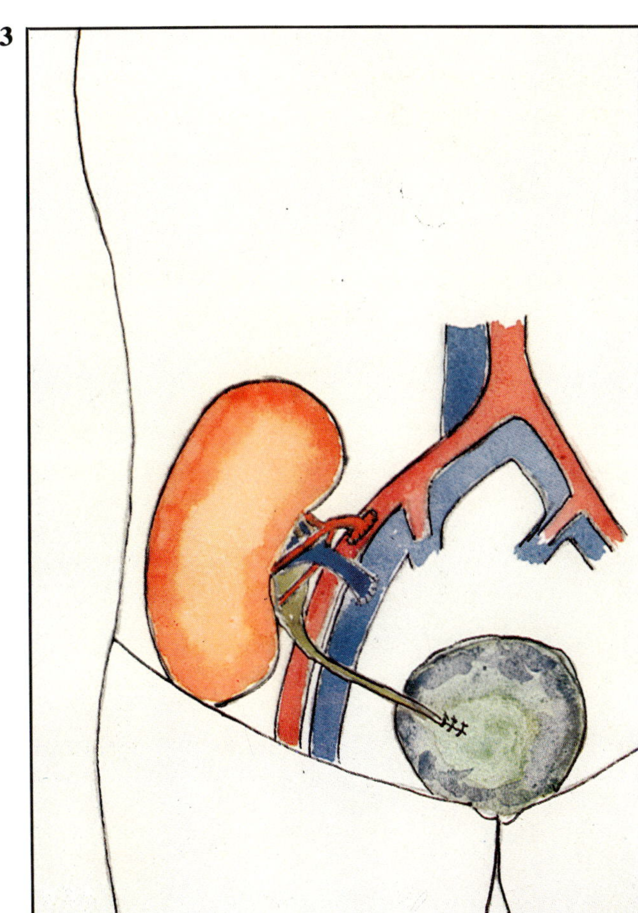

33 Diagram of completed recipient operation. The kidney is in the extraperitoneal plane in the right iliac fossa. The renal artery with a Carrel patch is anastomosed end-to-side to the proximal portion of the external iliac artery, the renal vein end-to-side to the external iliac vein. The ureter is implanted into the bladder near the dome with a submucous tunnel.

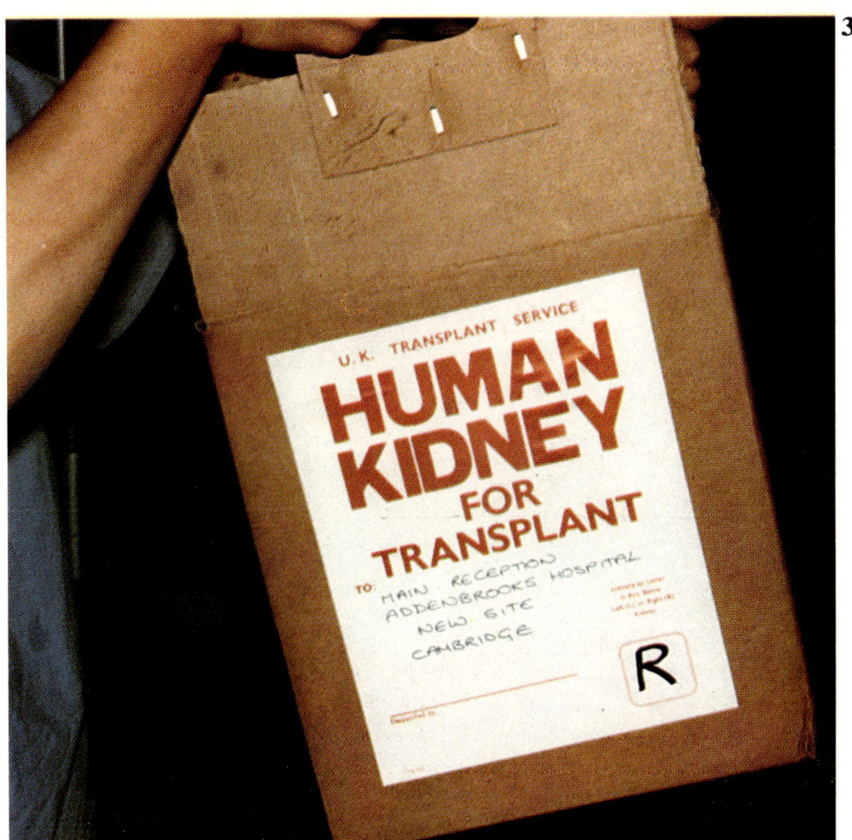

34 The kidney transport box. The box is marked clearly 'Human Kidney for Transplant' and the side, in this case R for right. Anatomical details are written on a form stating whether the blood vessels, ureter, and kidney itself are normal. Any deviations from the usual anatomy are detailed.

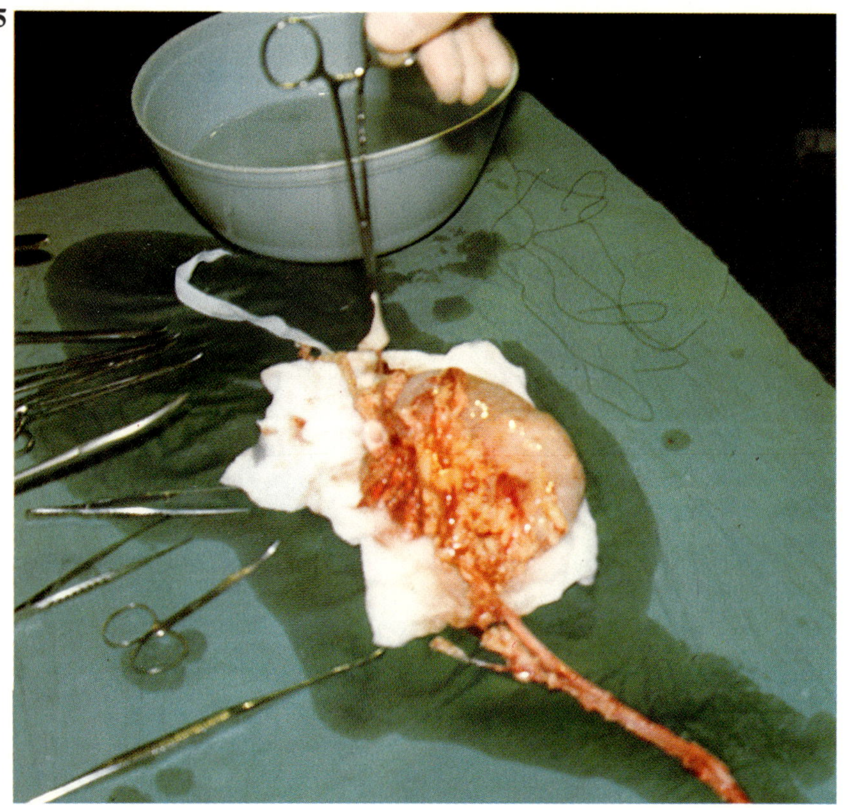

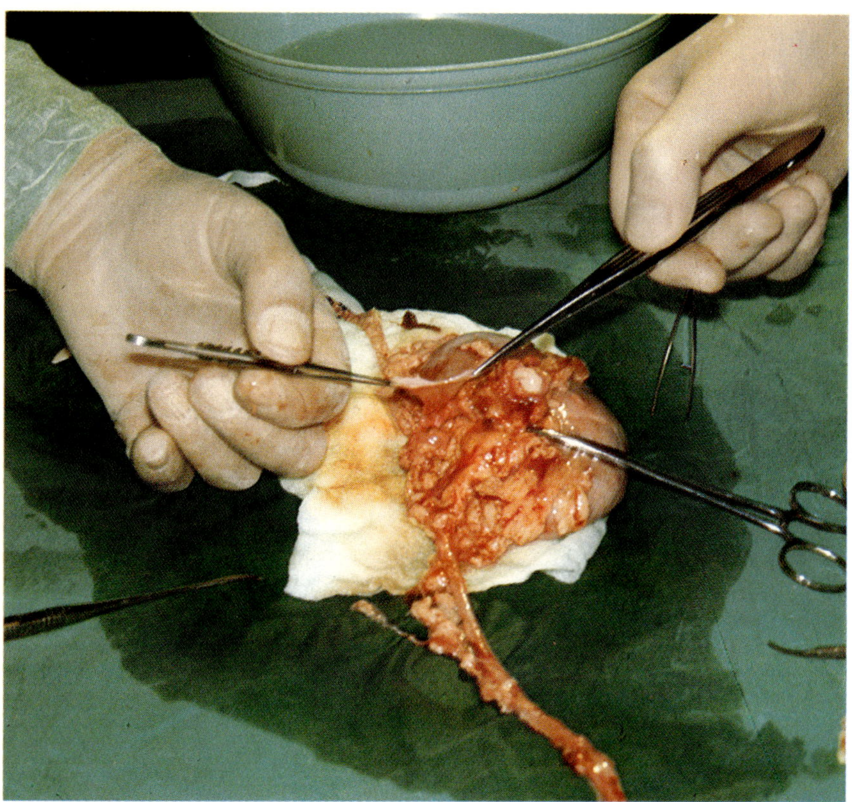

35 Inspection and assessment of graft anatomy. If the kidney has come from another hospital, no matter how close the working relationship is between the two institutions, the responsibility for the recipient belongs to the surgeon performing the transplant. The kidney is removed from ice before the operation starts on the recipient, so that the integrity of the main renal artery, vein and ureter can be confirmed and any anomalies noted. Serious abnormalities would preclude the kidney transplant operation. The kidney is removed from the transport box and, on a sterile table arranged like a workbench, a careful inspection is made and any necessary trimming or repairs are effected. This figure shows the renal artery in the centre with a small cuff of aorta around it.

36 Inspection of the renal vein shown stretched between two forceps. The ureter runs towards the middle of the bottom of the frame.

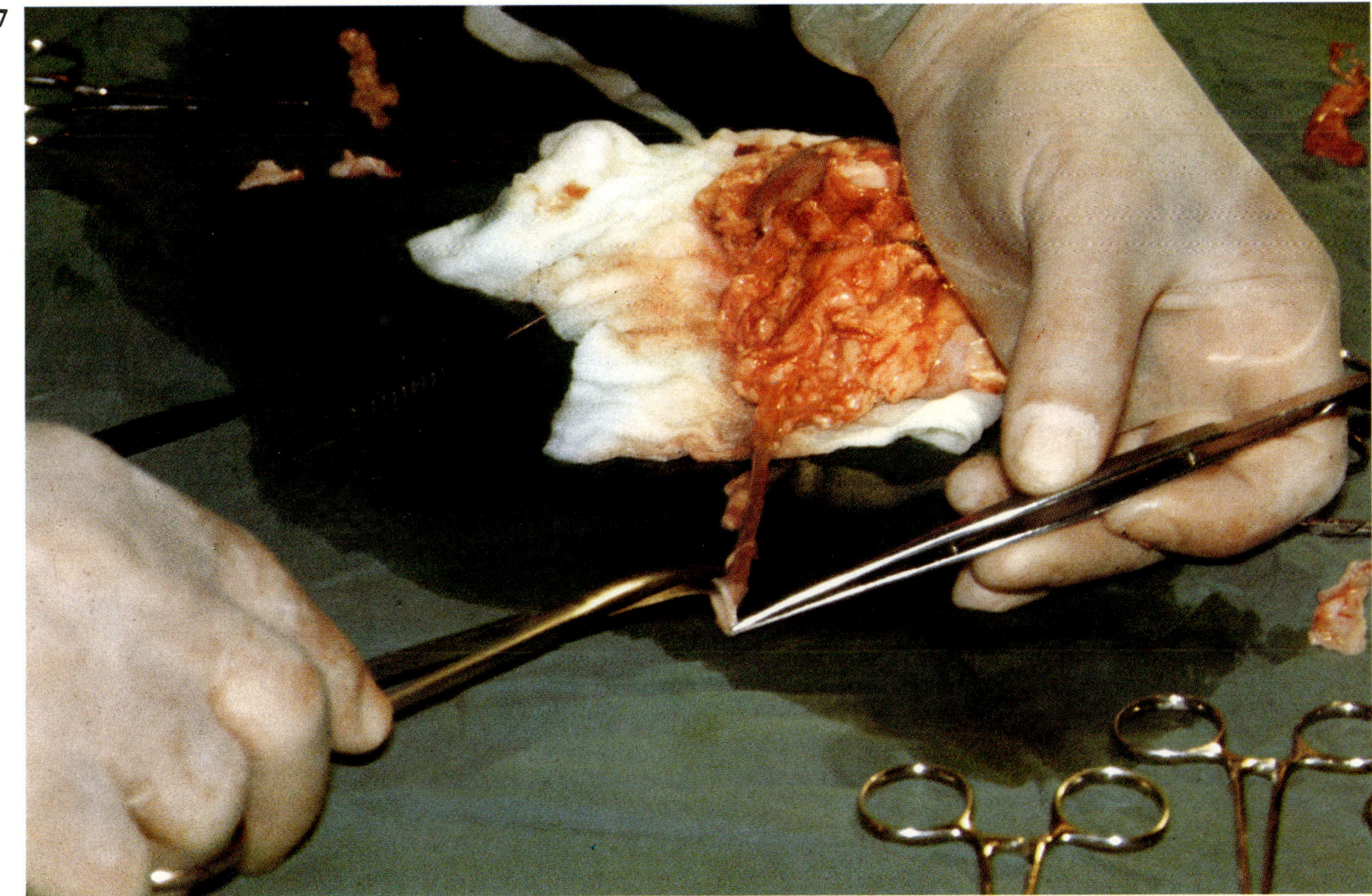

37 **Trimming of the ureter.** The ureter has been cut back so that the blood supply to the distal cut end is not endangered. An incision is made 8mm along one edge to give a spatulated appearance to provide an oblique anastomosis, wider than could be achieved if the ureter was cut transversely.

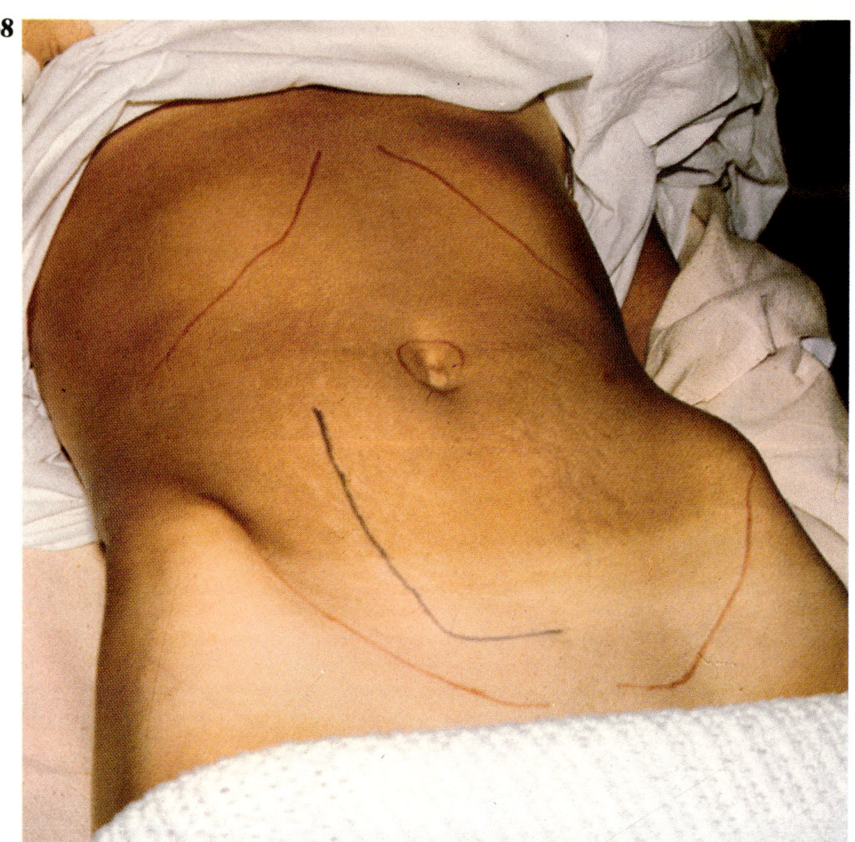

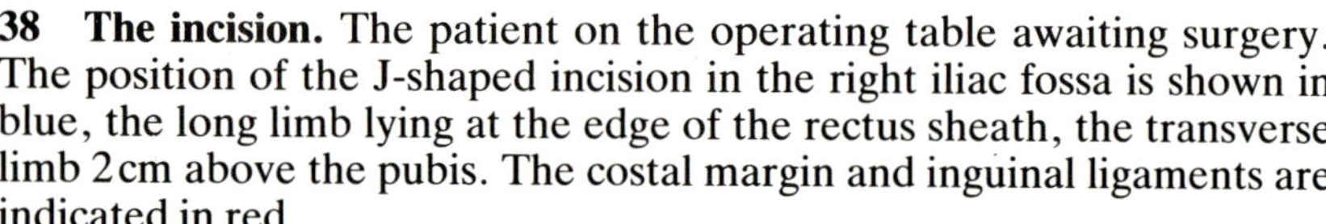

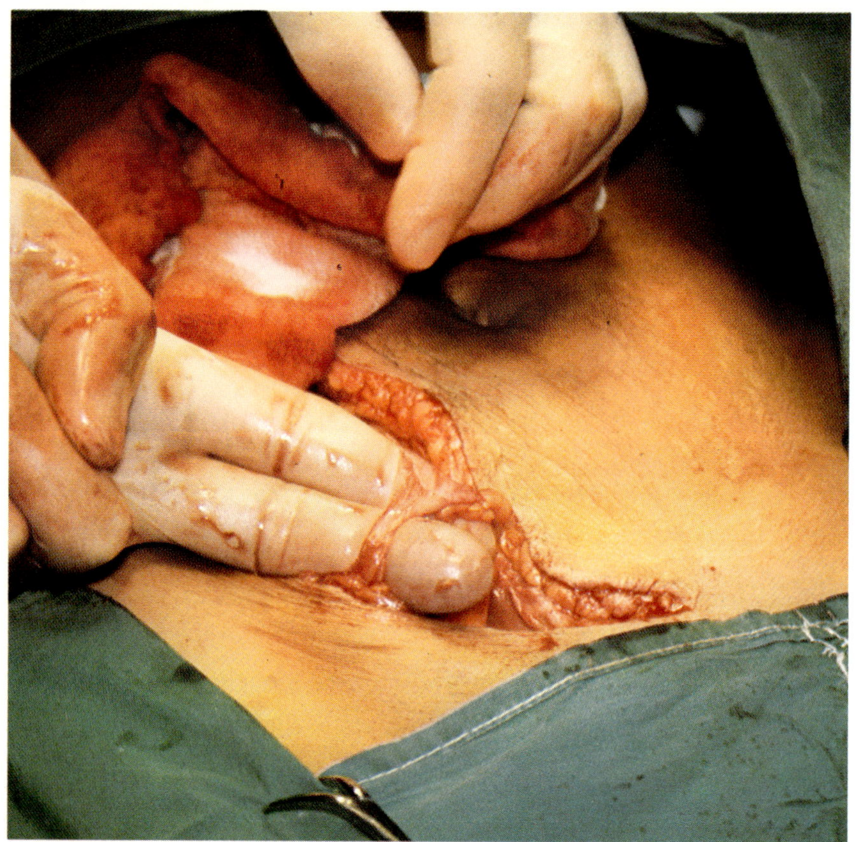

38 The incision. The patient on the operating table awaiting surgery. The position of the J-shaped incision in the right iliac fossa is shown in blue, the long limb lying at the edge of the rectus sheath, the transverse limb 2 cm above the pubis. The costal margin and inguinal ligaments are indicated in red.

39 The round ligament displayed over the fingertips. The incision has been made through the skin, subcutaneous tissues and musculofascial layers. The inferior epigastric vessels have been ligated with catgut and divided.

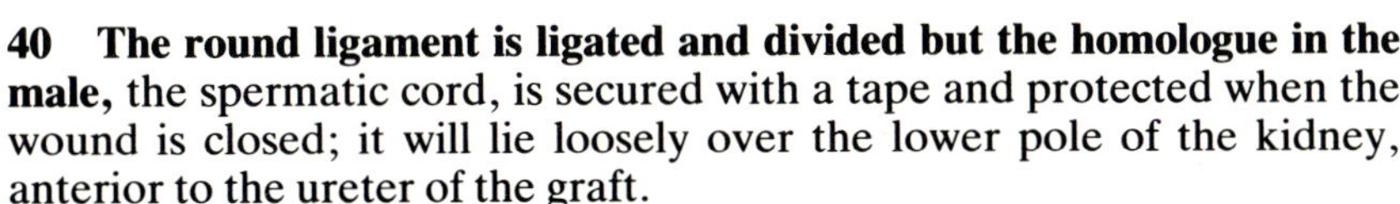

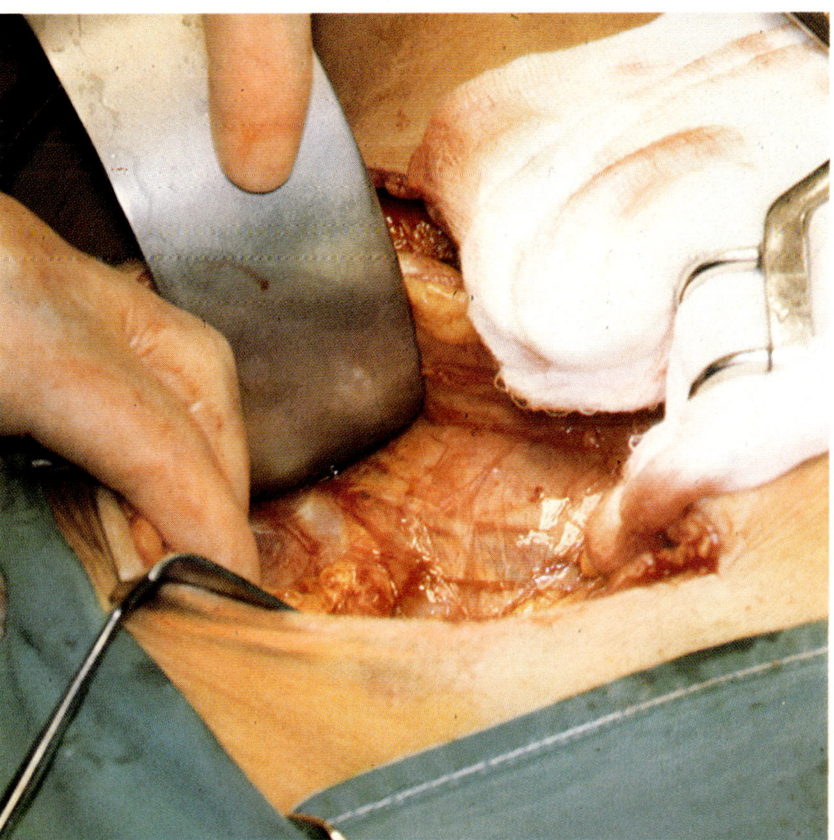

40   The round ligament is ligated and divided but the homologue in the male, the spermatic cord, is secured with a tape and protected when the wound is closed; it will lie loosely over the lower pole of the kidney, anterior to the ureter of the graft.

41   Dissection in the extra-peritoneal plane. A self-retaining Balfour retractor has been inserted; one assistant is holding a Deaver superiorly and another a Langenbeck retractor laterally.

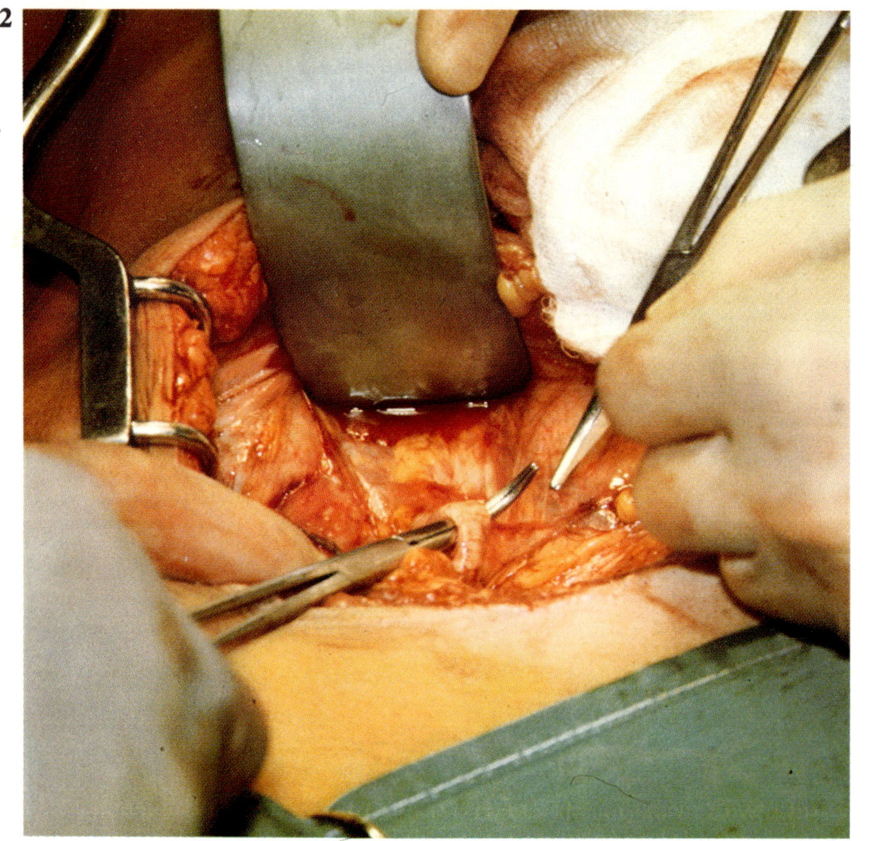 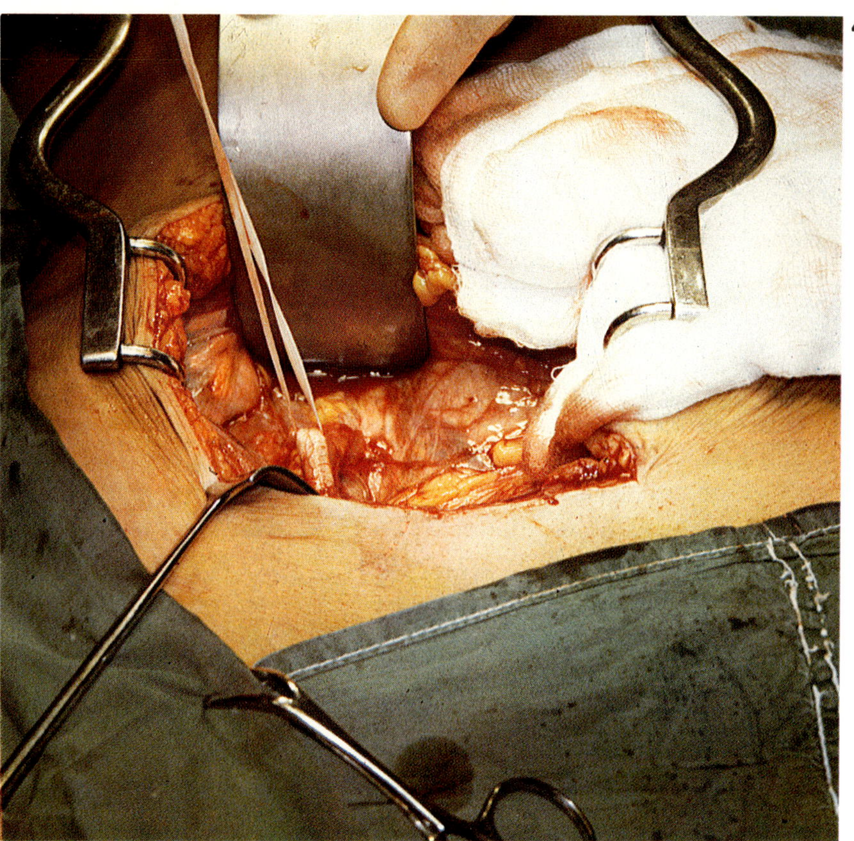

42   Identification and control of the external iliac artery. A right angle forceps passes beneath the external iliac artery ready to receive a tape.

43   The tape in position around the external iliac artery.

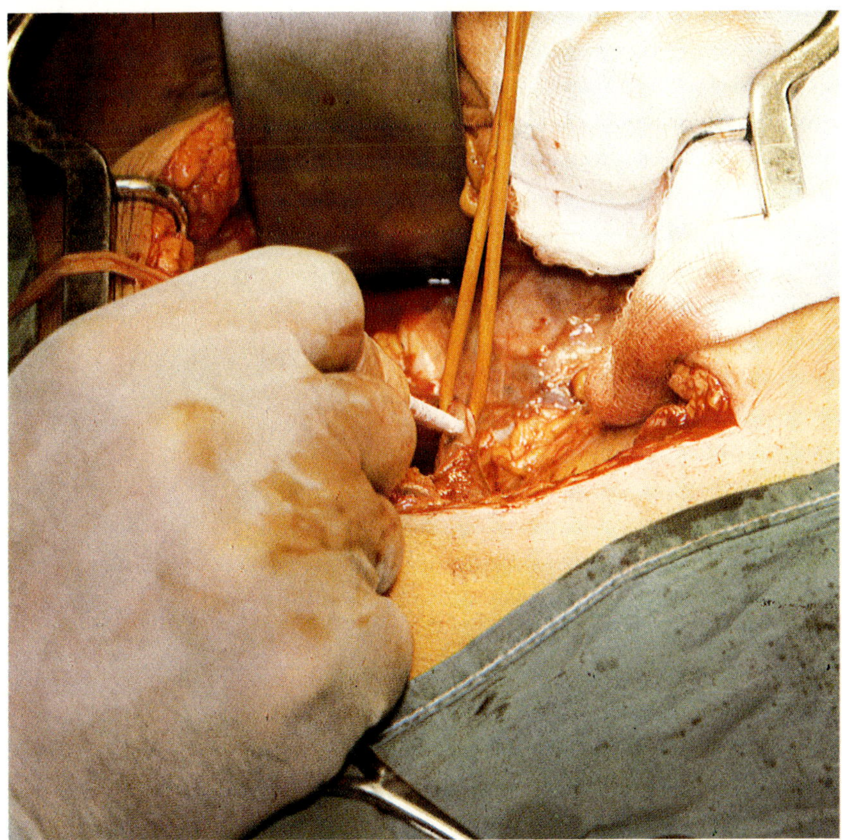

44 **A soft rubber sling is passed around the external iliac vein.** The vein is on the right, the artery on the left of the figure.

45 **Distal clamping of the external iliac vein.** The vessel is held up by the rubber sling towards the leg and the bulldog clamp shown with the blades covered with white cloth is about to be applied to the vein just above the inguinal ligament.

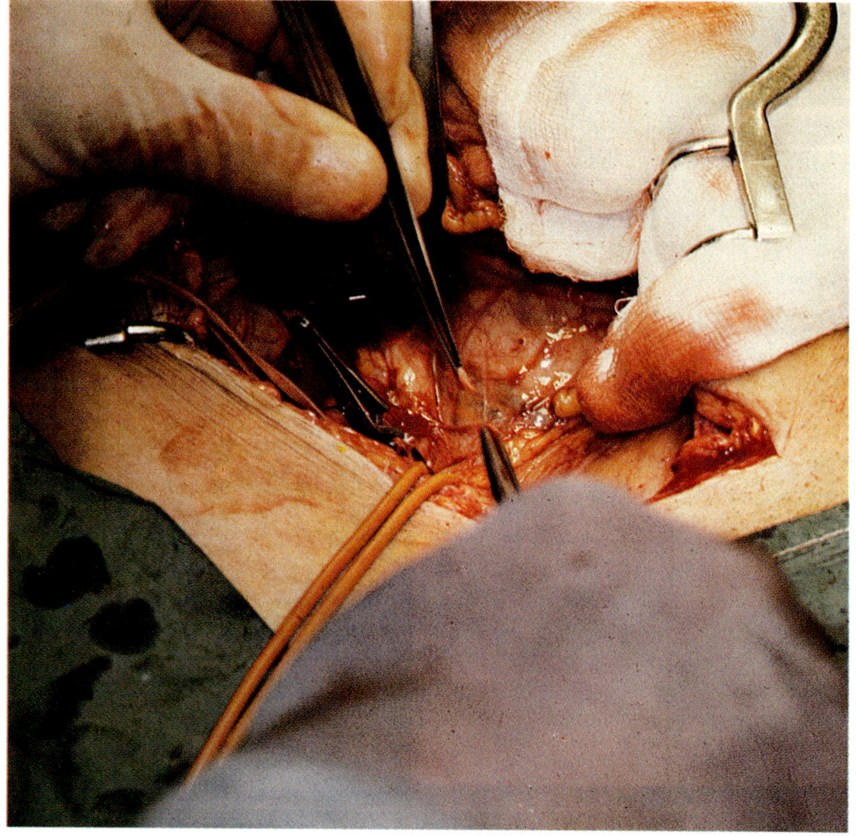

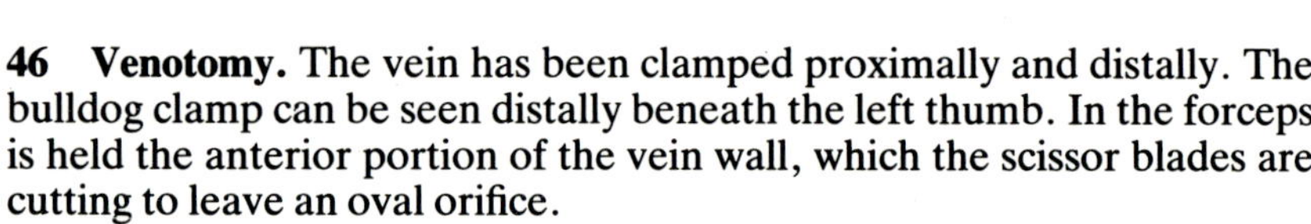

46   **Venotomy.** The vein has been clamped proximally and distally. The bulldog clamp can be seen distally beneath the left thumb. In the forceps is held the anterior portion of the vein wall, which the scissor blades are cutting to leave an oval orifice.

47   **The oval portion of vein removed in the forceps.**

48 Diagram of stages for end-to-side anastomoses of both artery and vein.

a) A double-ended atraumatic 5/0 prolene stitch is used; the first stitch from within the lumen of the incision in the recipient vessel and the end of the donor vessel.

b) Using traction with a strabismus hook at the opposite extremity of the donor vessel, stitching is begun from within, the first stitch passed from outside the recipient vessel to within the lumen. The other end of the suture is held out of the way with a bulldog clip.

c) The posterior wall is nearly completed, being sewn over and over from within. If there is a tendency to inversion then eversion mattress sutures are inserted.

d) Commencement of the anterior wall, again usually over and over with an occasional mattress if necessary using the other end of the atraumatic stitch. The first end has been held out of the way with a bulldog clip.

e) The anterior wall is nearly completed. Traction with a strabismus hook makes the suturing easy.

f) Anastomosis completed.

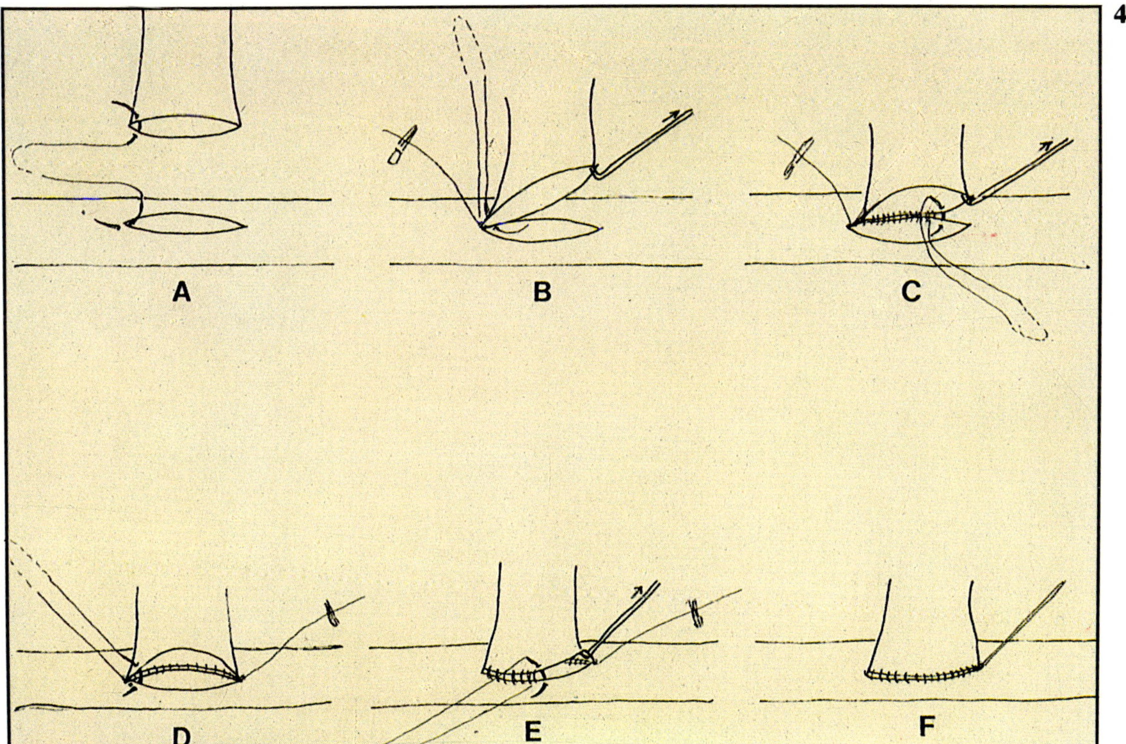

49 The oval orifice in the front of the external iliac vein. The lumen has been irrigated with heparinised saline and there is no bleeding. A 5/0 double-ended prolene suture has been inserted through the upper proximal extremity of the venous orifice.

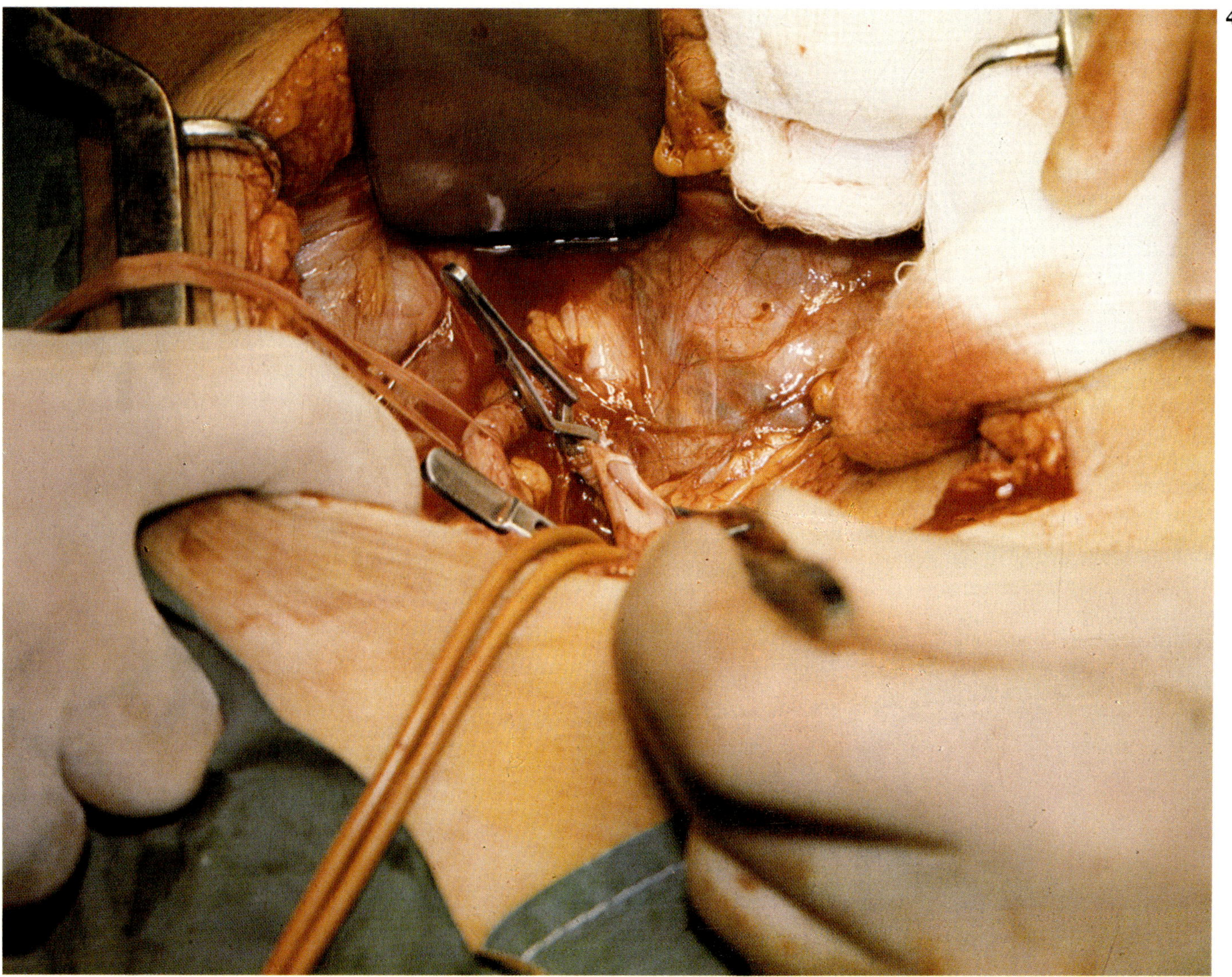

50   Close-up view of first 5/0 prolene stitch being inserted. The atraumatic forceps in the vein lumen facilitate the placing of the suture.

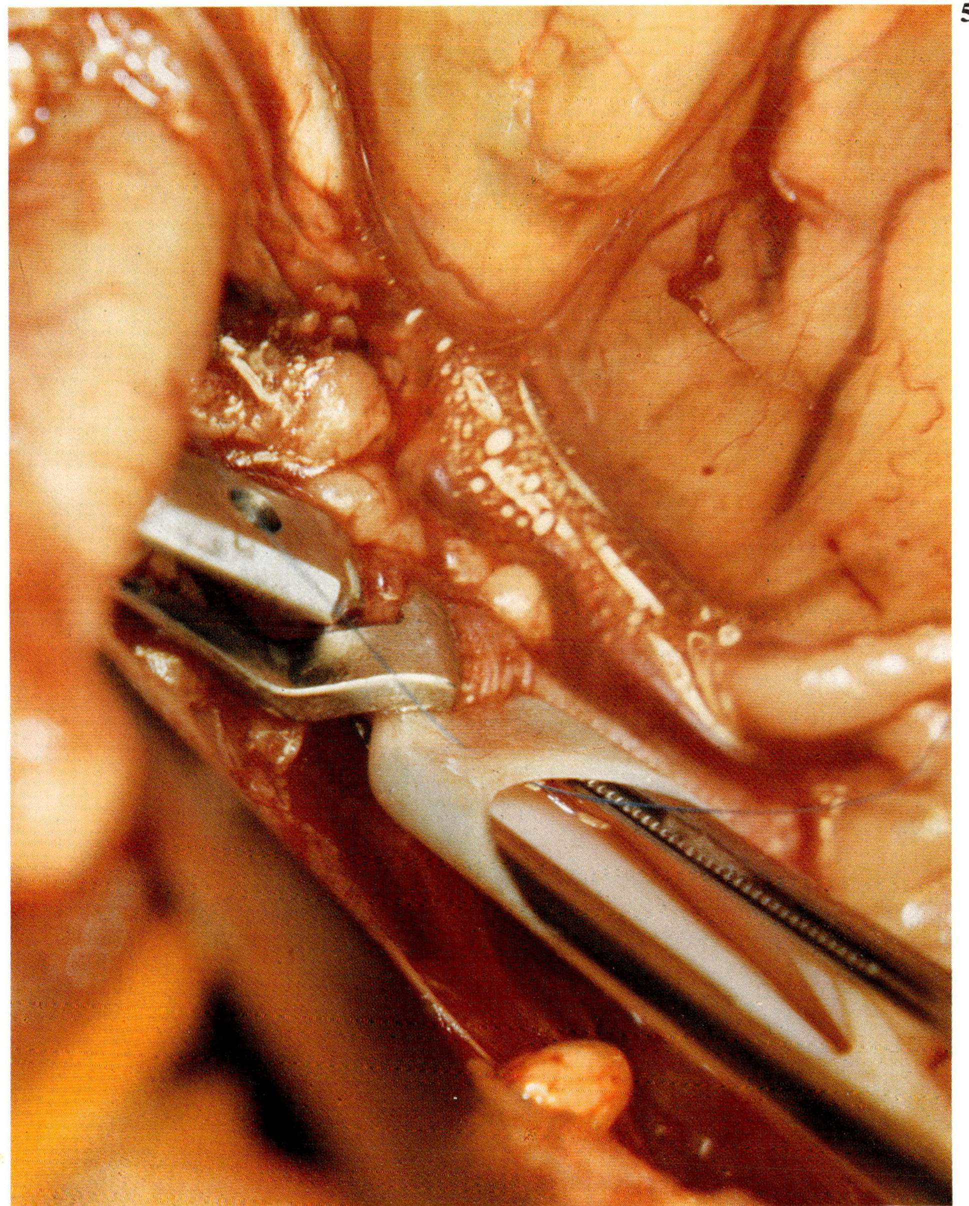

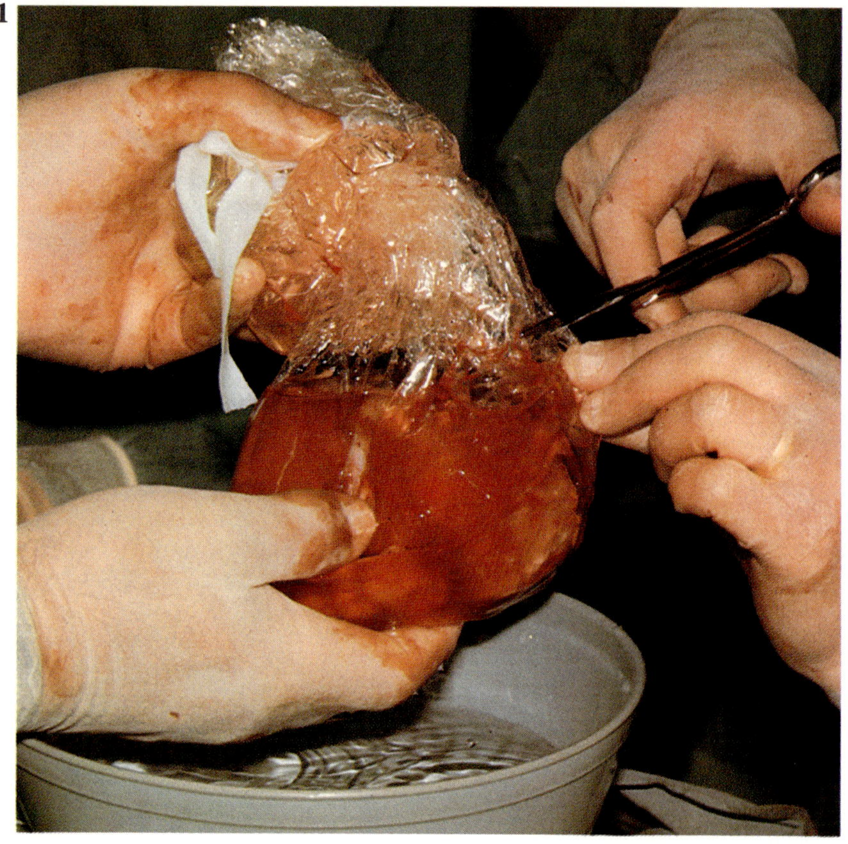

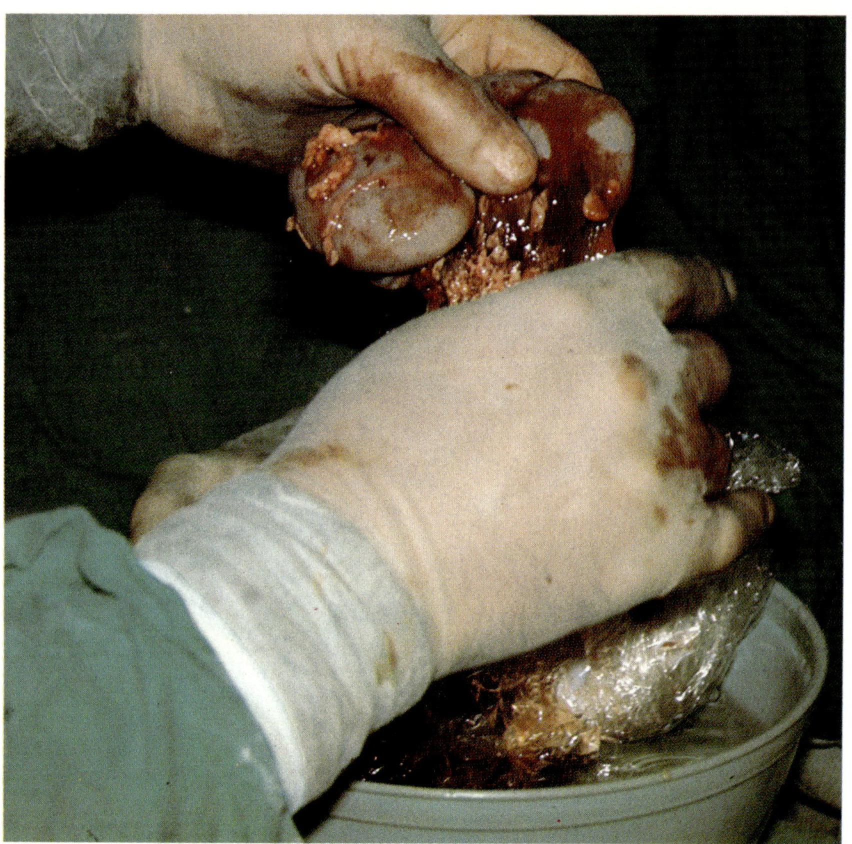

51 Removal of the kidney in its plastic bag. The inner bag containing the kidney has been removed from the outer bag, the outside of which was not sterile. The inner bag is sterile both outside and inside and is being opened with a pair of scissors.

52 The cold kidney is gently removed from the bag.

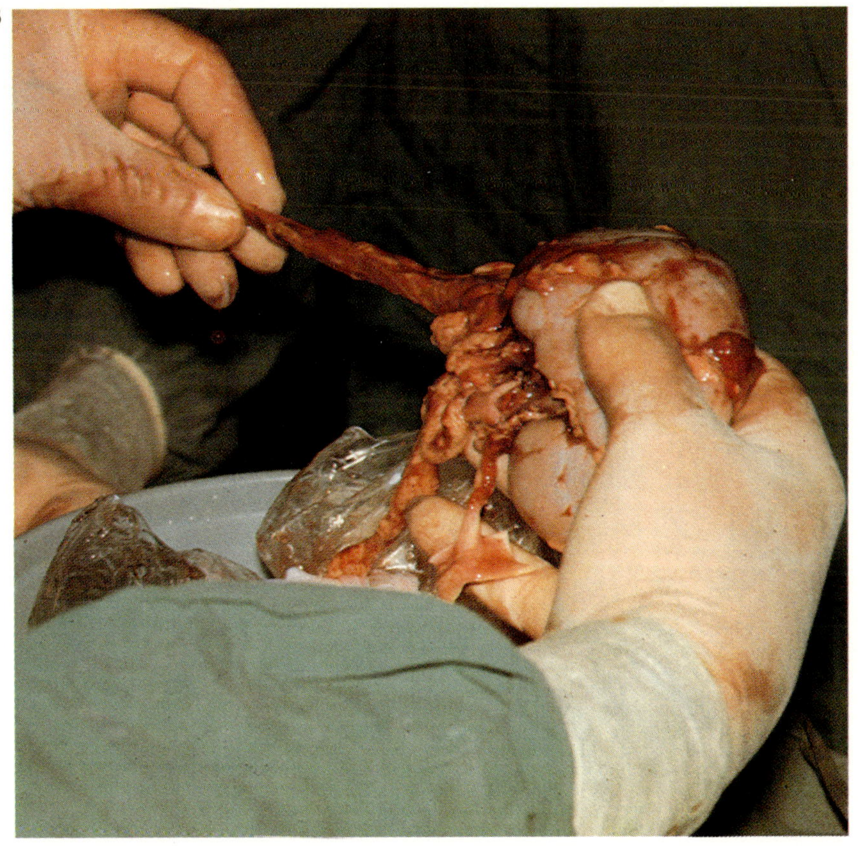

53 The graft anatomy is displayed. The ureter is held in the left hand and the kidney in the right. The renal artery with a patch of aorta is lying on the tip of the finger.

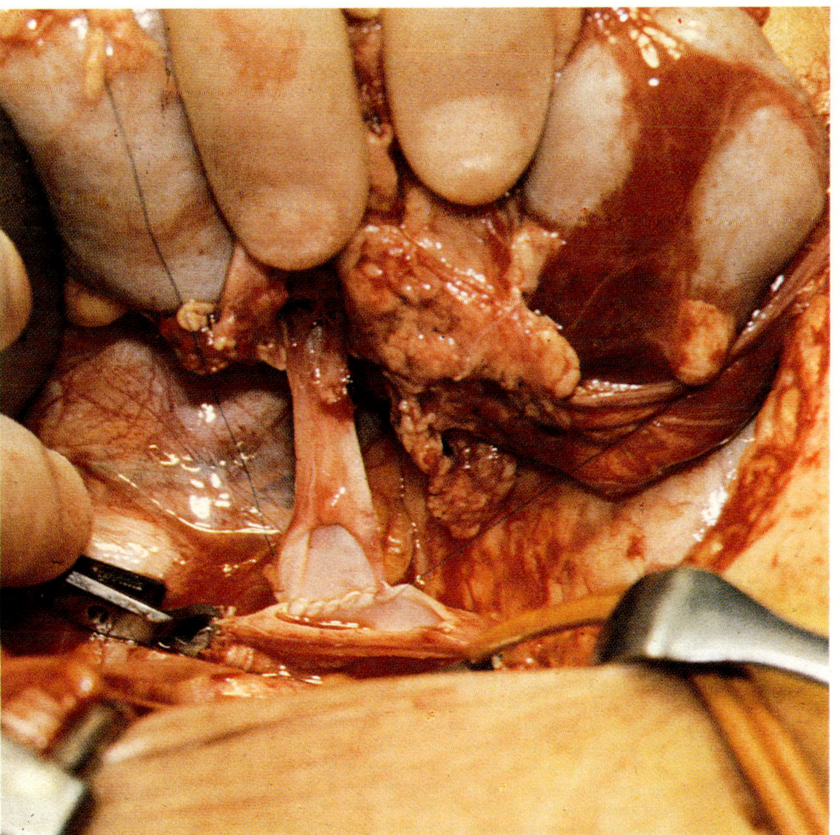

54 Orientation of the kidney. The ureter is shown to the right passing upwards. The renal vein is in the middle passing vertically downwards to the orifice in the external iliac vein. The medial posterior wall of the anastomosis has been sutured from the inside from proximal to distal. The posterior wall is two-thirds completed in this picture.

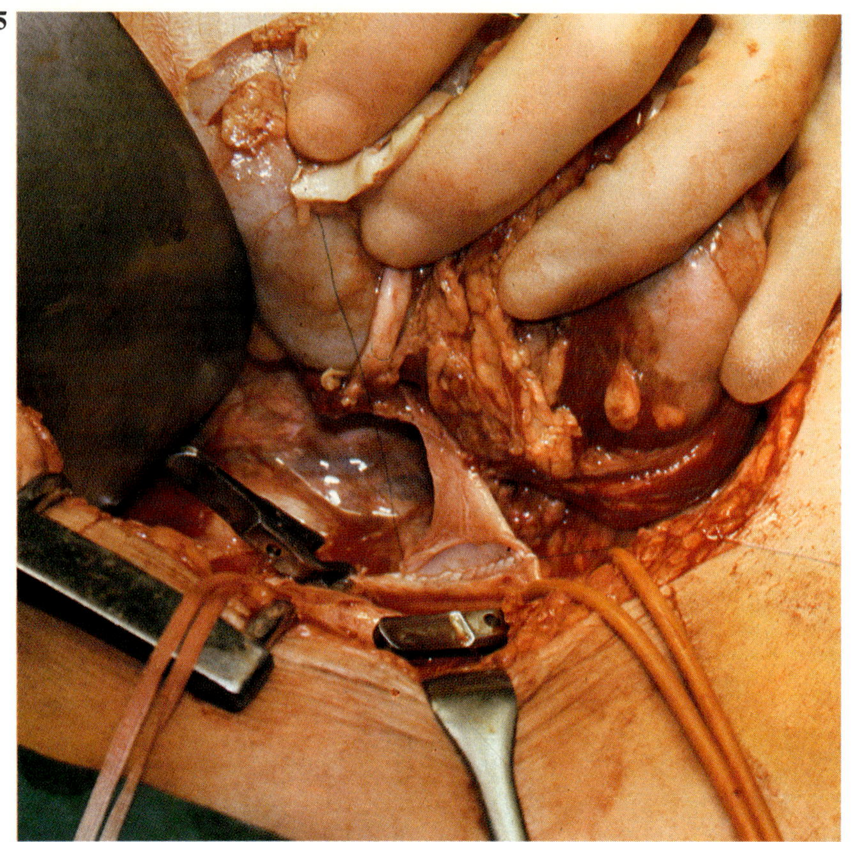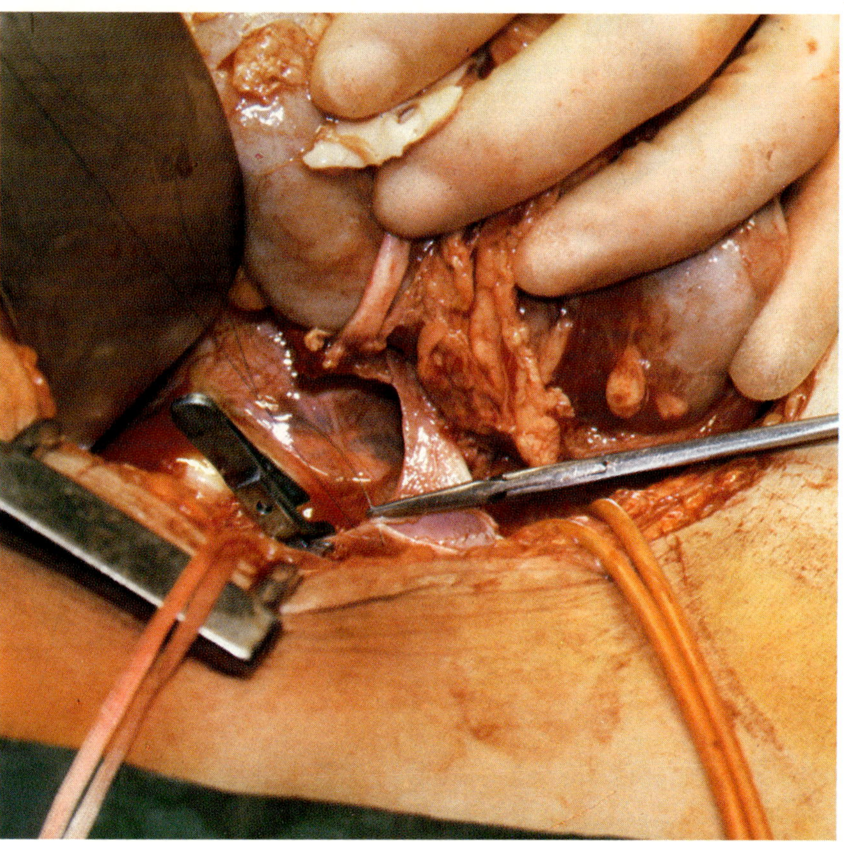

55 **The posterior wall of the venous anastomosis is completed.** The anterior wall anastomosis is about to be commenced from proximal to distal. The Carrel patch of aorta with the renal artery is seen between the index and middle fingers of the assistant's hand above.

56 **Commencement of the anterior wall venous anastomosis.**

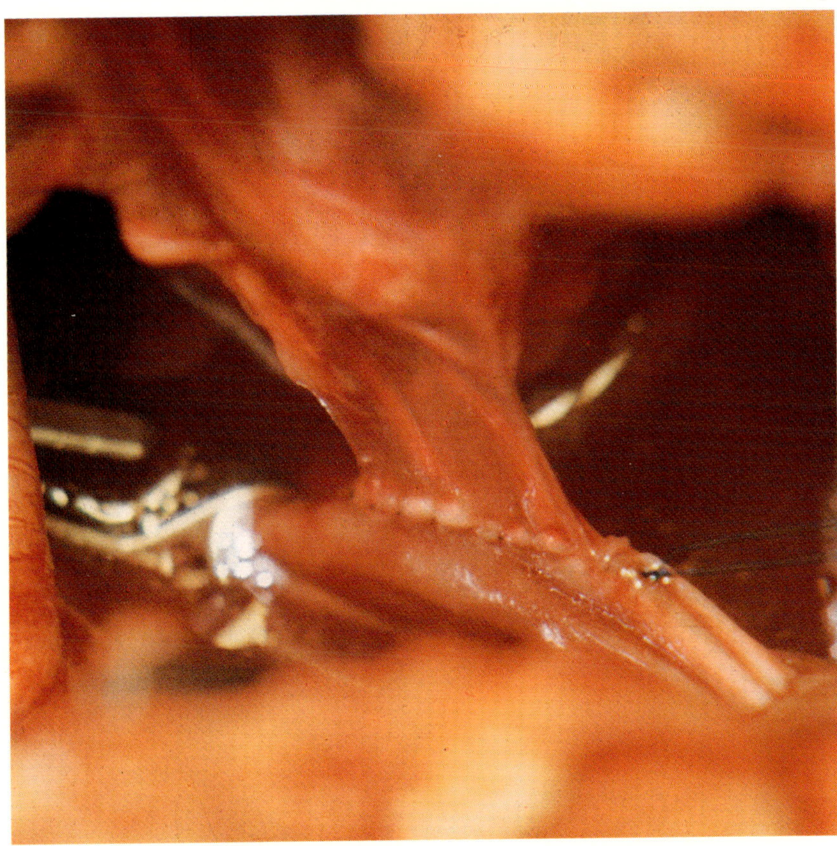

57 **Completion of the anterior wall venous anastomosis.** The renal vein is joined end-to-side to the external iliac vein, which is still clamped and controlled with a rubber sling distally.

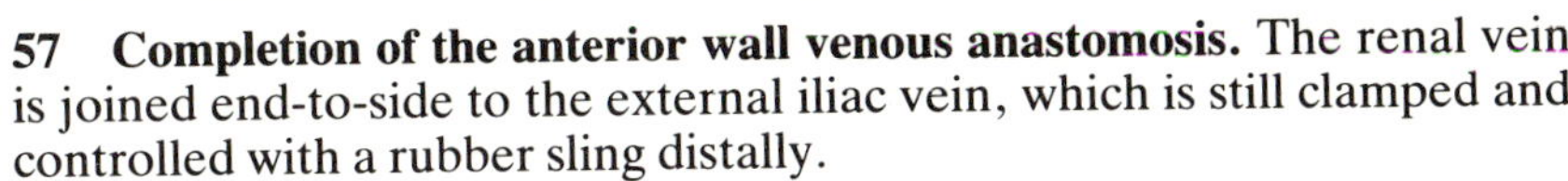

58 **Close-up of completion of anterior wall of venous anastomosis.**

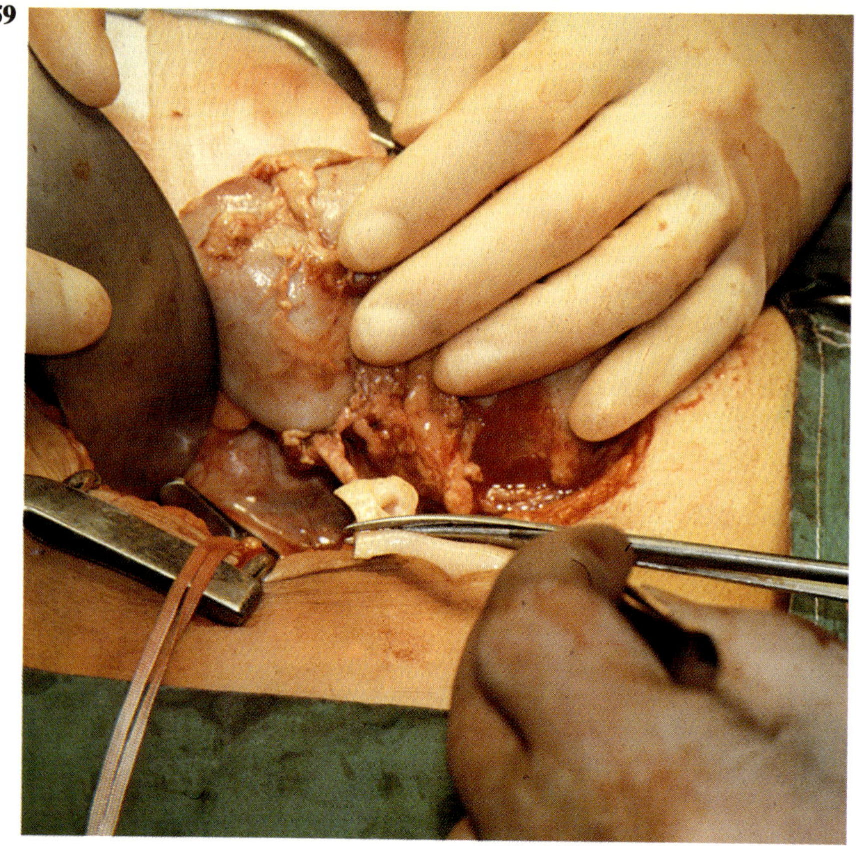

59 Preparation of the Carrel patch of aorta.

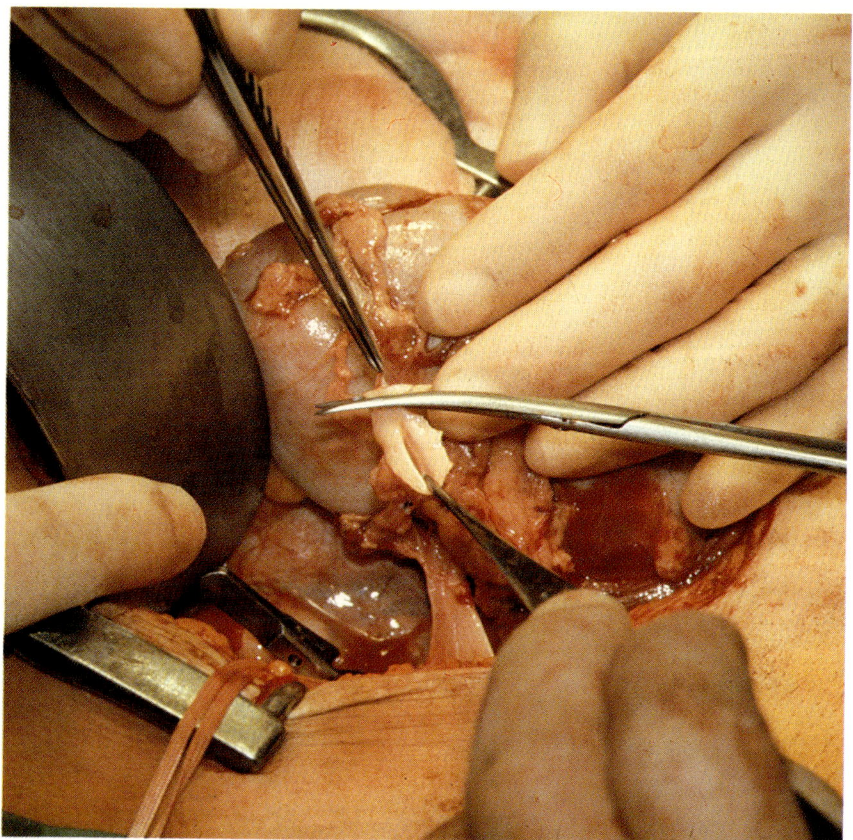

60 Trimming of arterial patch continues.

61 The arterial patch completed.

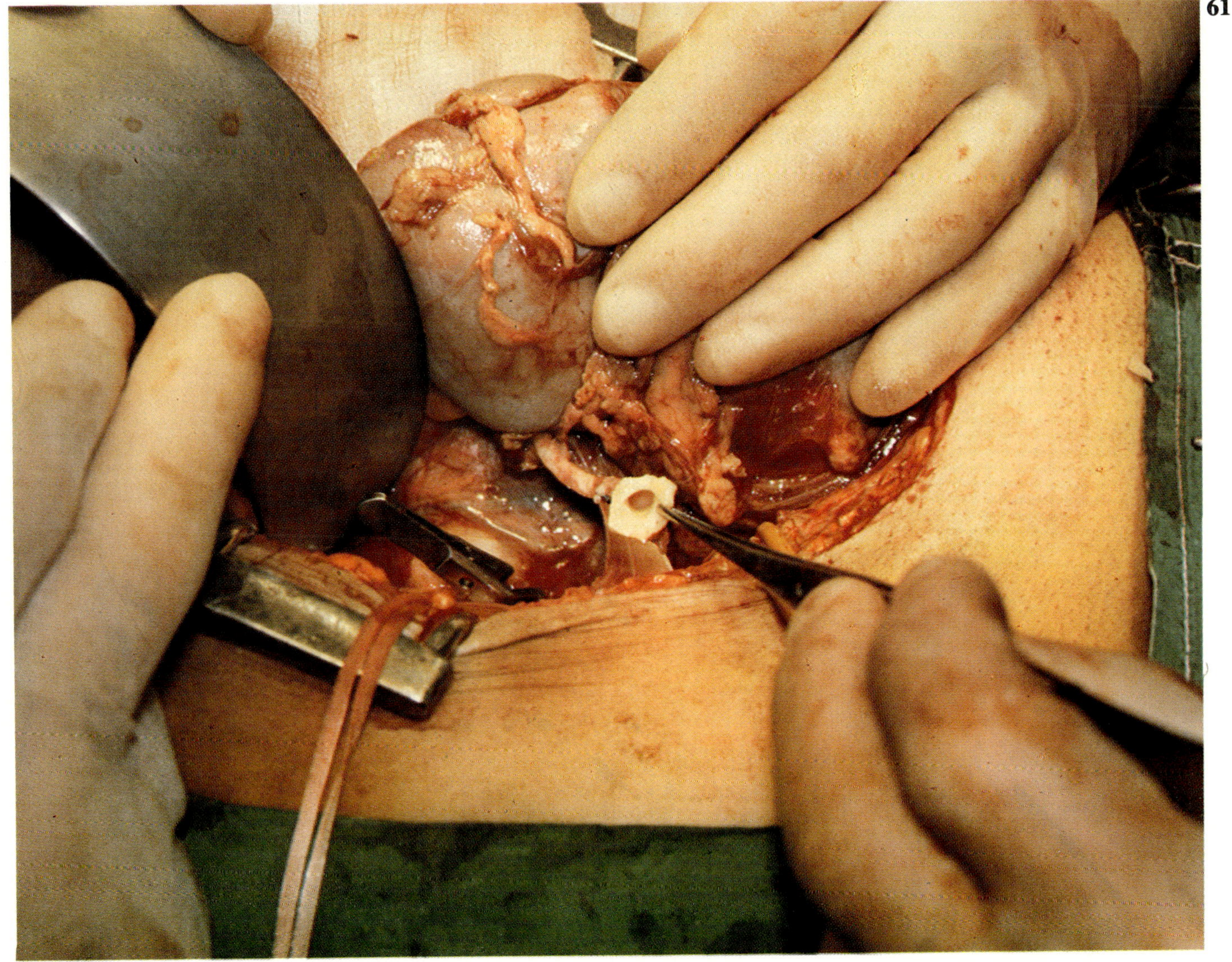

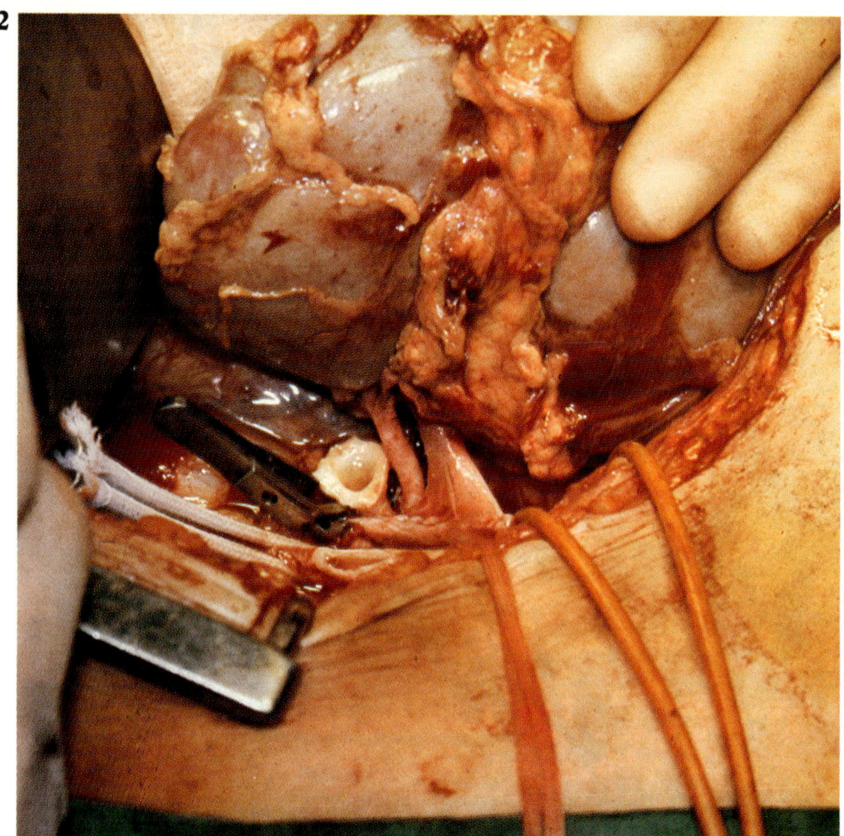

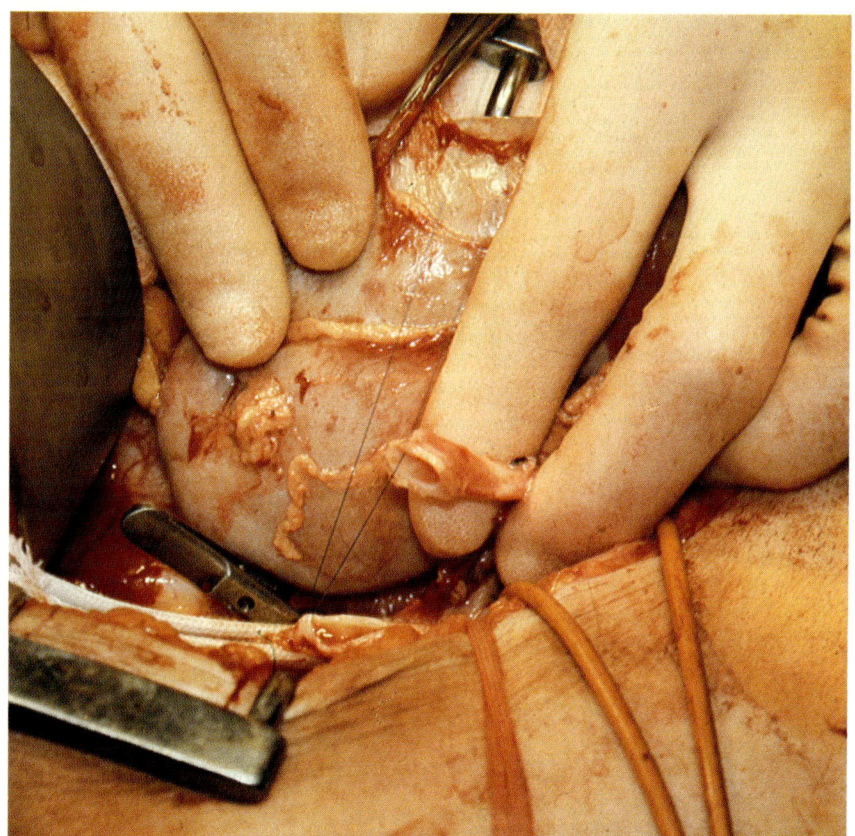

62   Clamping of the external iliac artery. A Crafoord clamp above and a bulldog clamp below, the latter cannot be seen. An oval orifice has been cut by scalpel incision and scissors trimming the front of the external iliac artery to receive the Carrel patch of aorta incorporating the renal artery.

63   The first 5/0 double-ended prolene stitch has been inserted through the proximal extremity of this orifice and the appropriate edge of the Carrel patch of aorta.

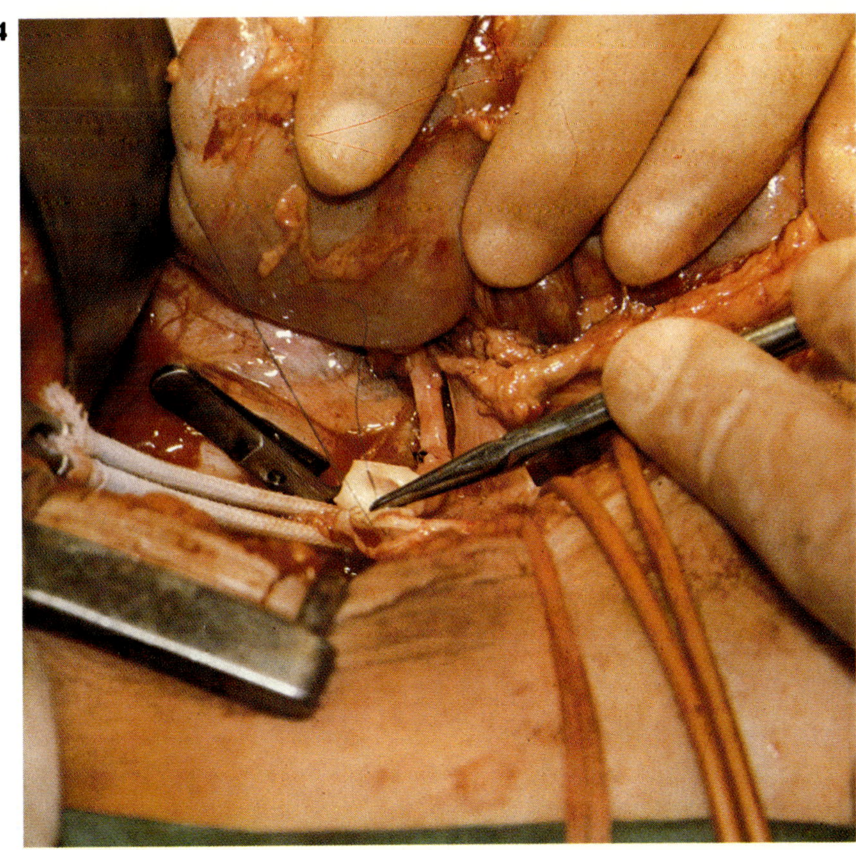

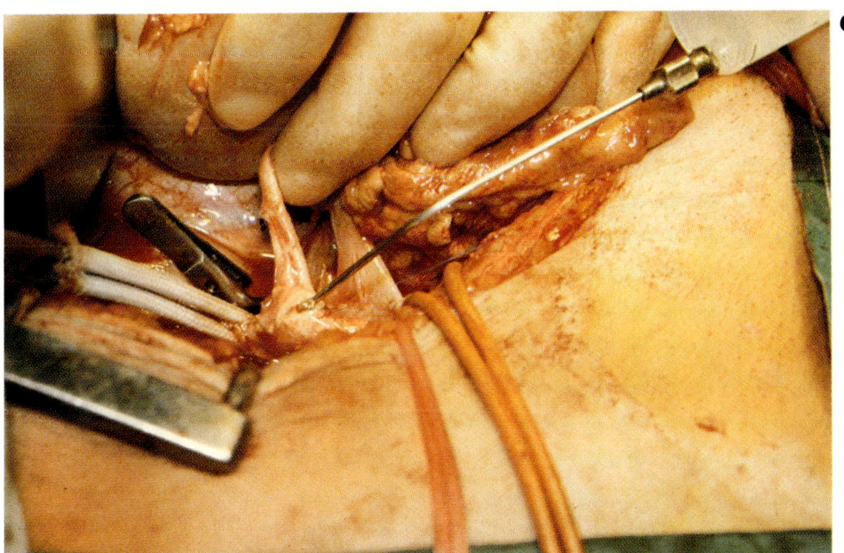

65 **The anterior wall of the arterial anastomosis.** This is two-thirds completed. The lumen is being irrigated with heparinised saline.

64 **The posterior wall of the anastomosis constructed from within.** A third of the length has been sutured.

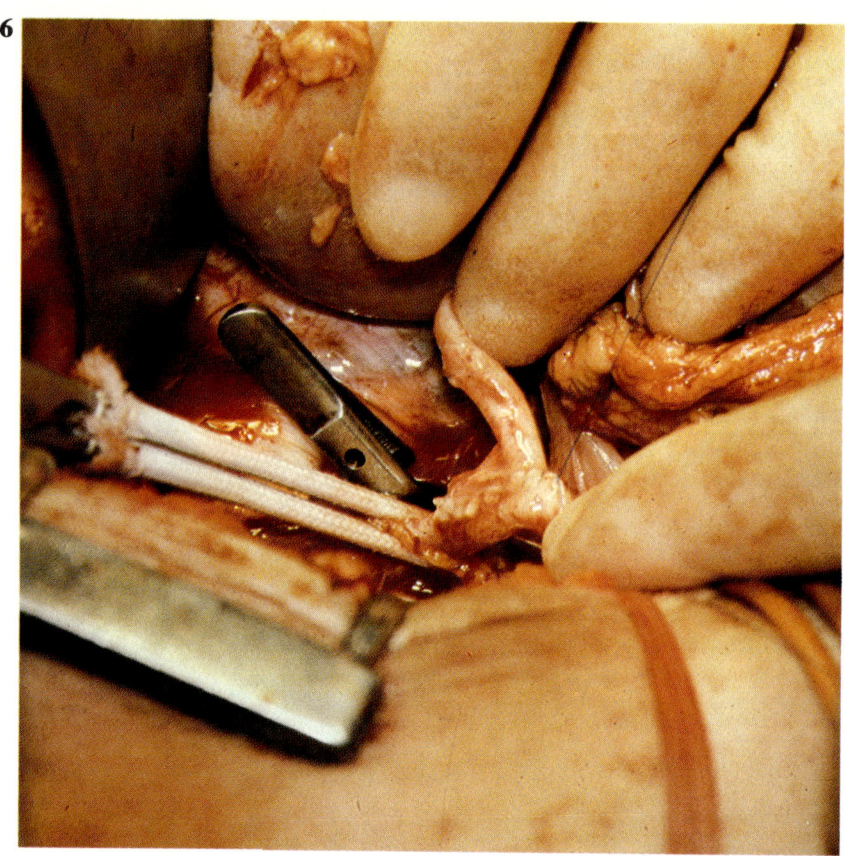

66 Anastomosis completed.

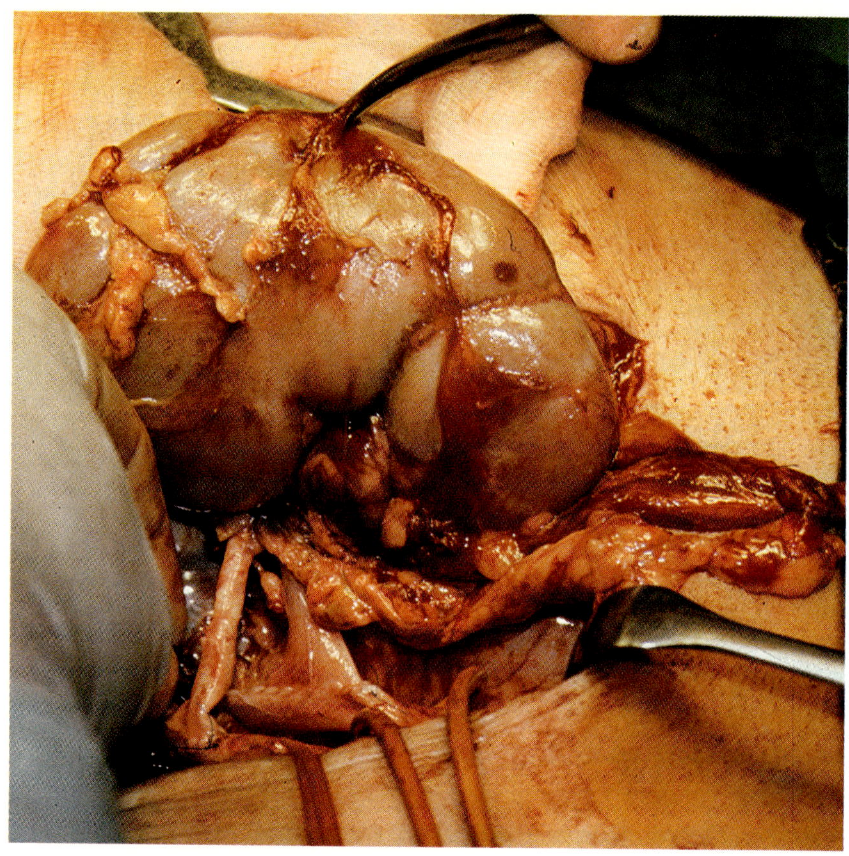

67 View of artery to the left, vein to the right. Both anastomoses completed. No blood yet through the kidney.

68 Vascular clamps removed. Both the artery and vein have filled with blood and the kidney has started to go pink.

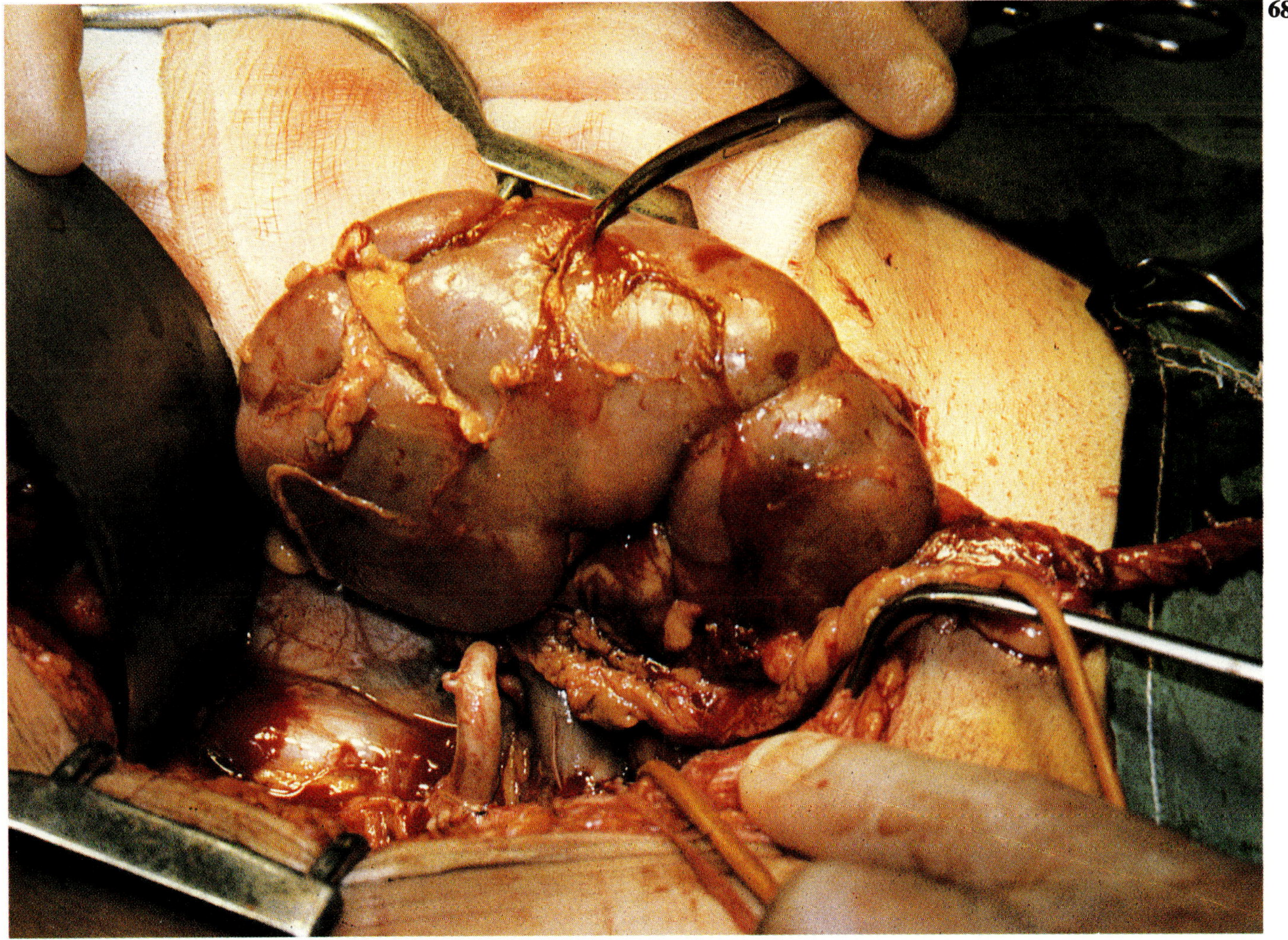

69 Further stage in re-vascularisation. The ureter appears well vascularised. Full flow now through the renal vessels.

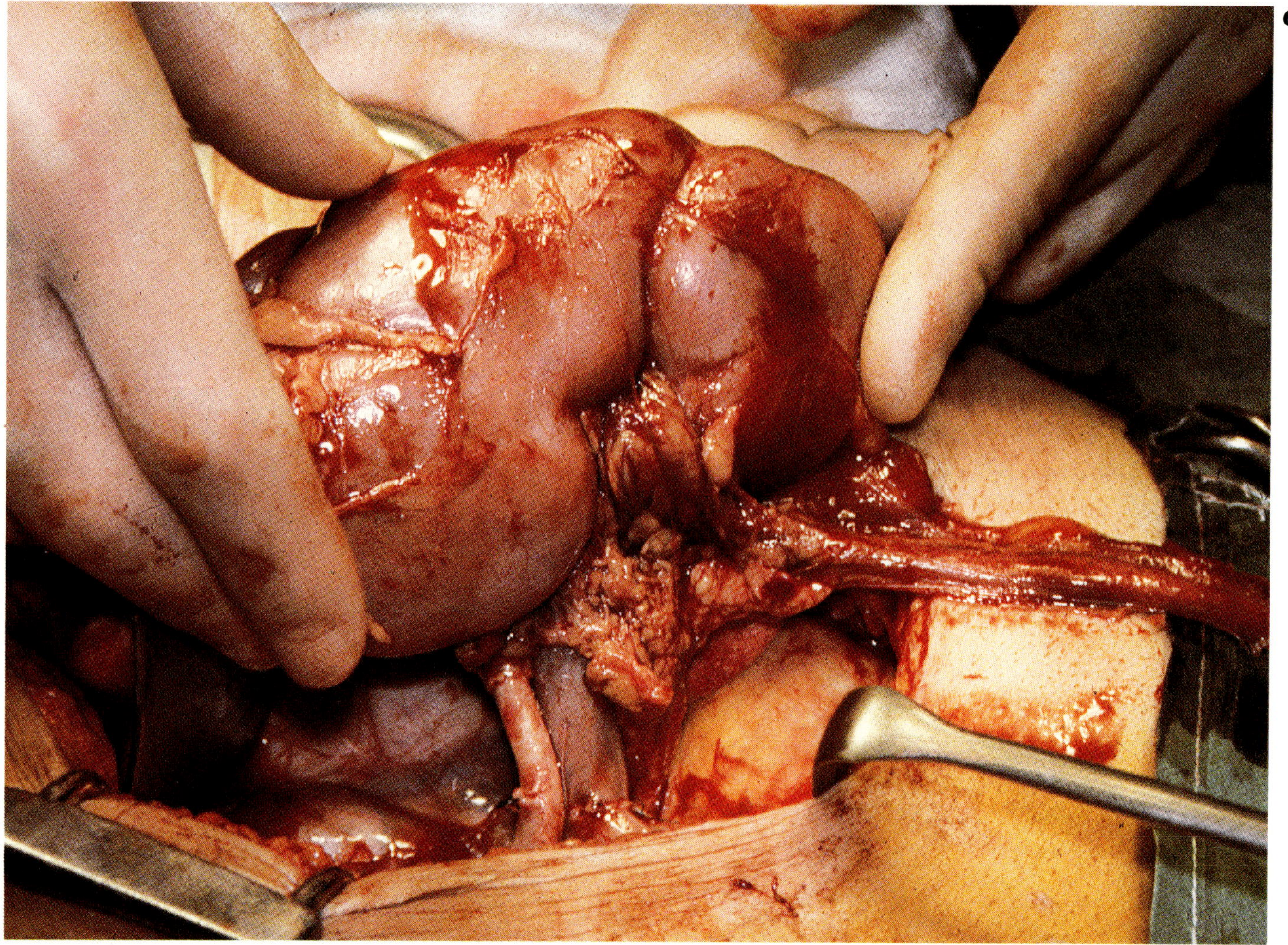

70 The artery has taken a curved configuration due to the systemic blood pressure being fully transmitted in it.

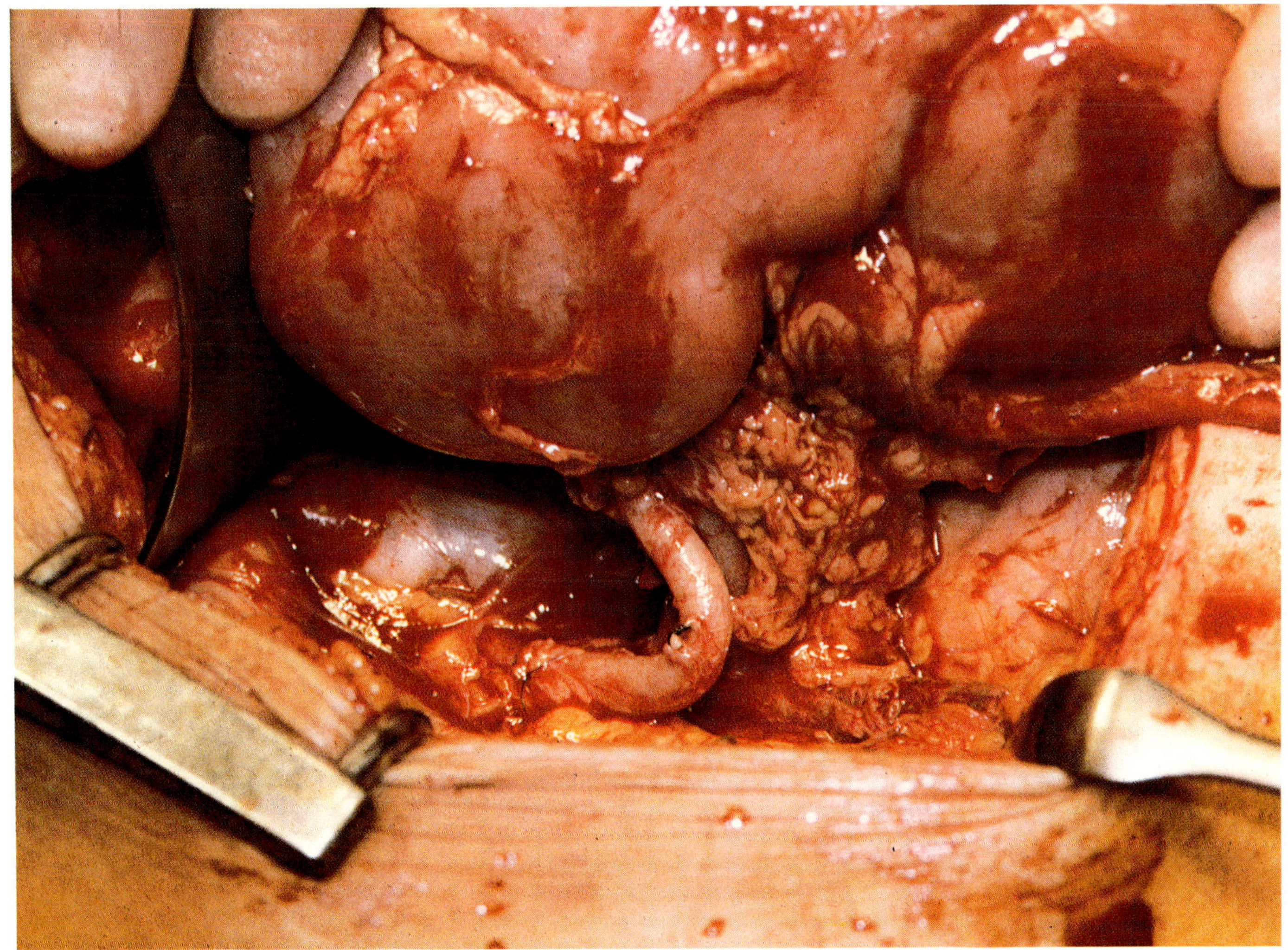

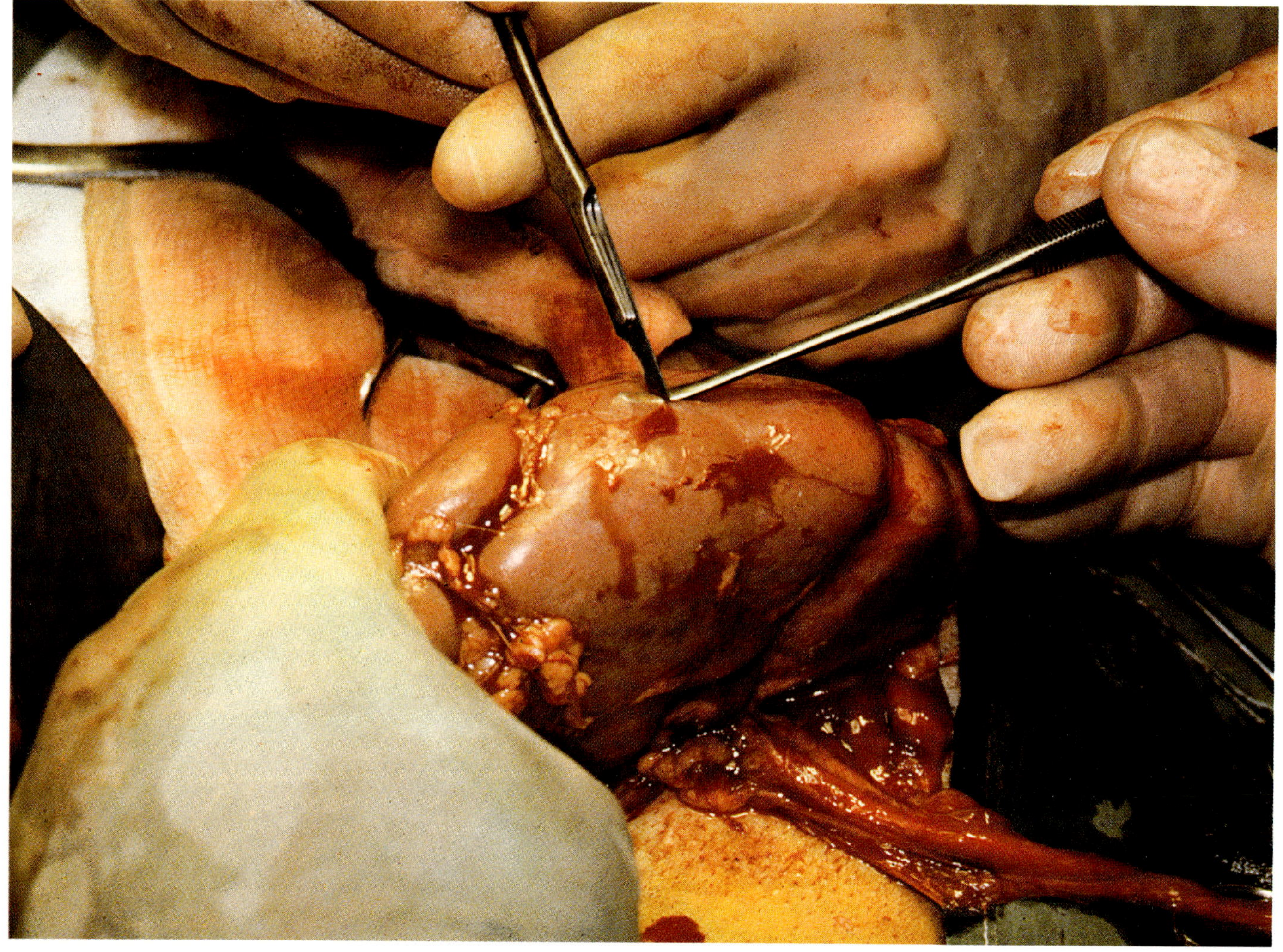

71 Capsulotomy. Through a small incision in the capsule; a Watson-Cheyne dissector is passed under the capsule and the capsule is incised. When the ischaemia period has been short, as in live kidney donation, capsulotomy is not performed.

Diagrams of stages in ureteric implantation

72 Incision of the end of the ureter for 0.8 cm to form a spatulated end for an oblique anastomosis.

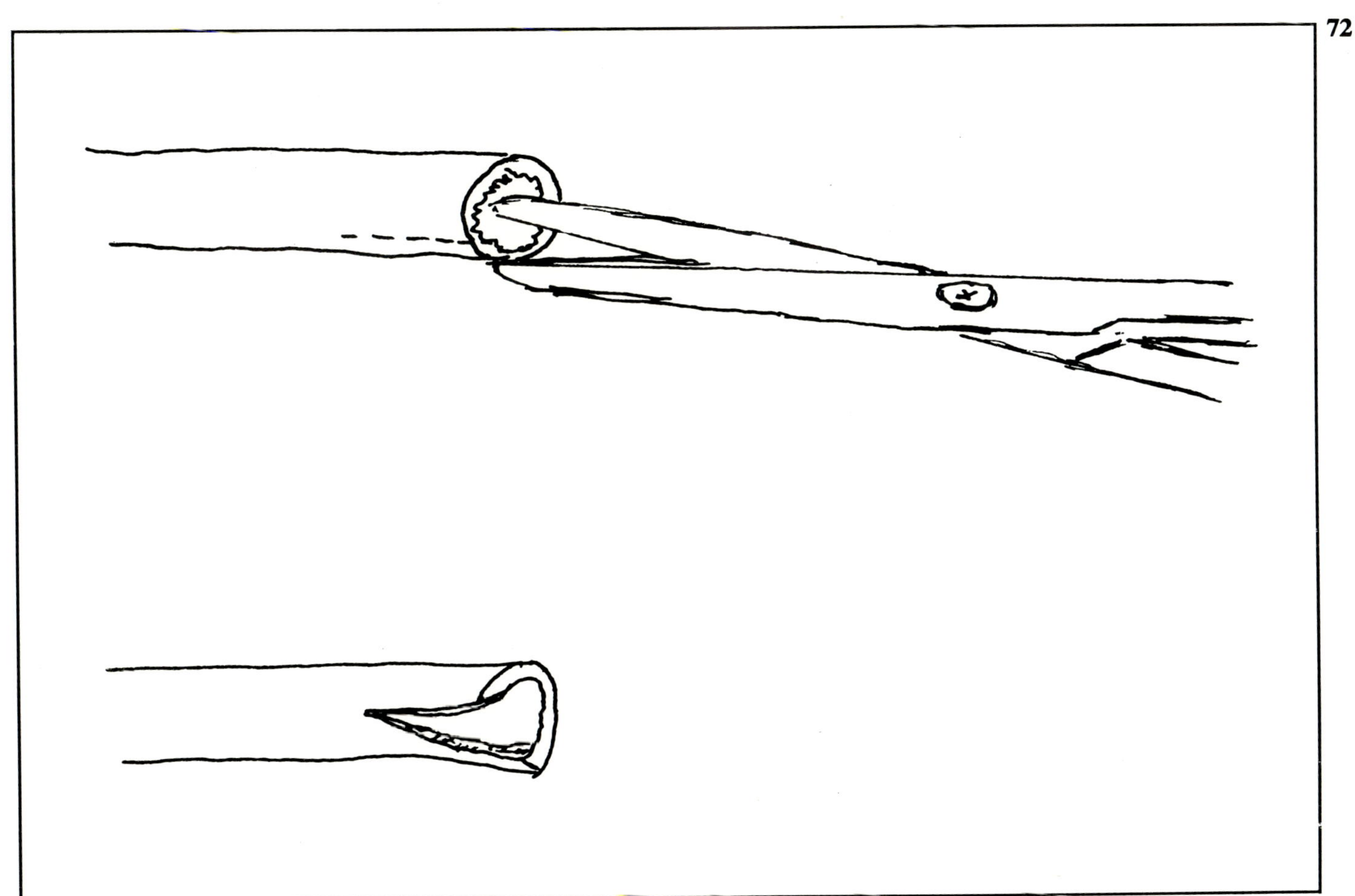

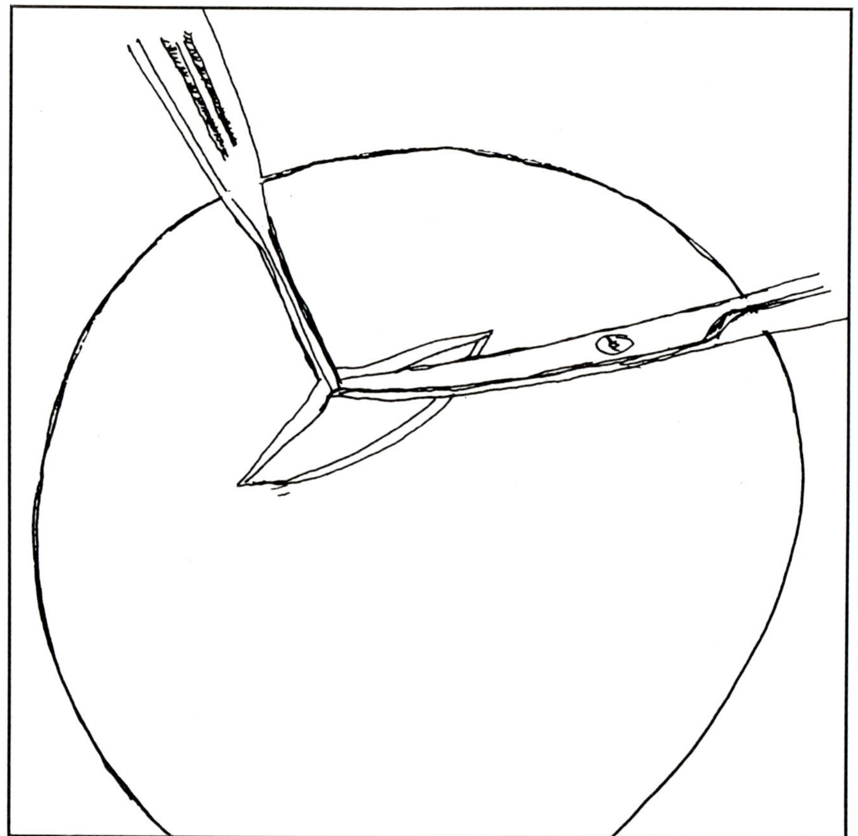

73 **Diathermy incision through the muscle of the bladder** for 2 cm in the supralateral aspect, until the mucosa pouts outwards. The bladder has been filled via a urethral catheter with sterile saline.

74 **Undermining of the muscle between it and the mucosa,** so that the muscle can be sutured over the ureter to form a valve after implantation.

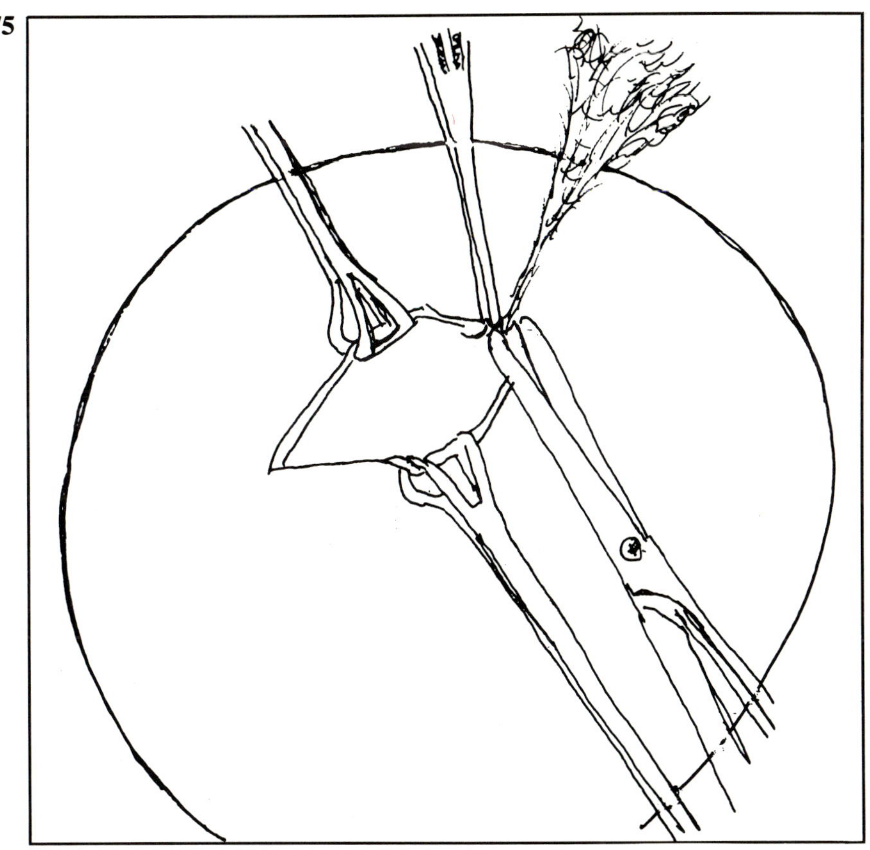

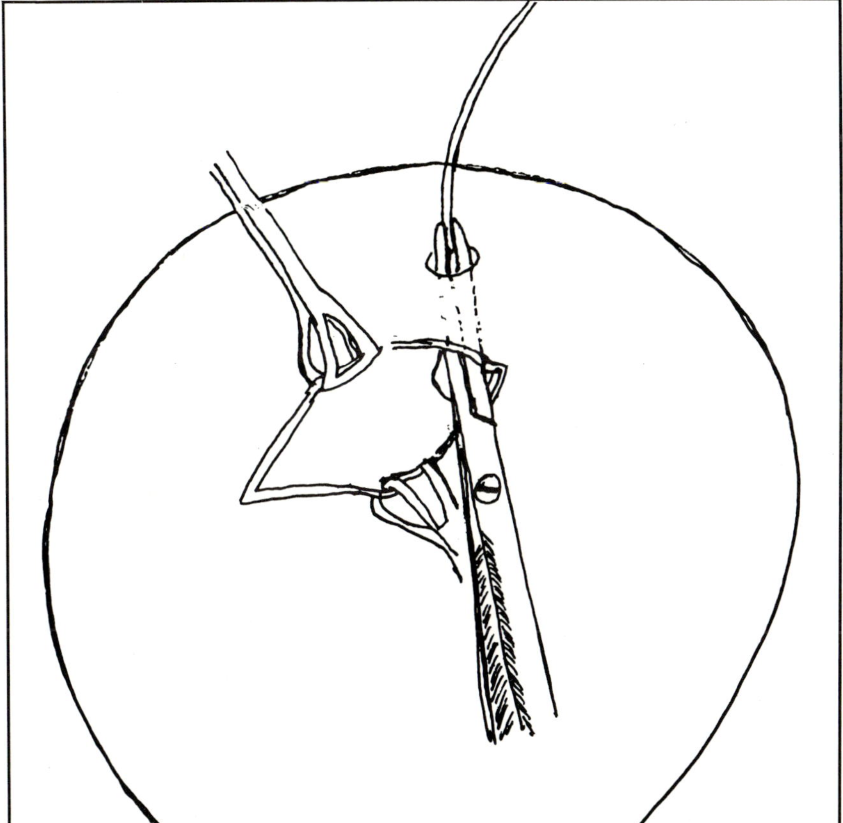

75 Incision of the bladder mucosa at the distal extremity. The sterile saline is shown escaping after the opening has been made. The bottle on the drip stand containing sterile saline, with which the bladder has been filled is now placed on the floor so that the saline is drained back into the bottle and does not flood the wound.

76 Insertion of a right angle forceps through the cystotomy. A knife incision is made over the tips of the forceps which then grasp a No. 6 Tizzard umbilical catheter. This is brought out through the initial incision.

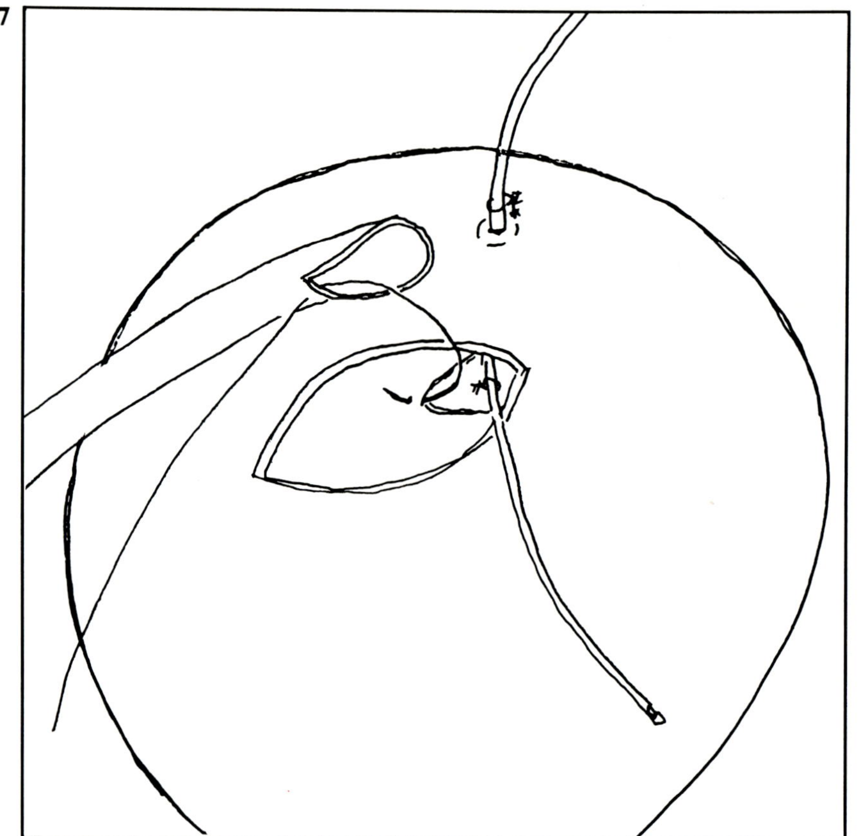

77   Shows the Tizzard catheter brought out through the incision in the bladder. It is secured to the bladder wall with a purse string 2/0 catgut suture. A 4/0 chromic catgut stitch has been tied around the catheter, and sutured to the bladder mucosa close to the anastomosis to discourage its dislodgement in the postoperative phase. The first 4/0 chromic catgut stitch has been inserted through the mucosa of the bladder and the end of the ureter near the apex of the cut in the ureter.

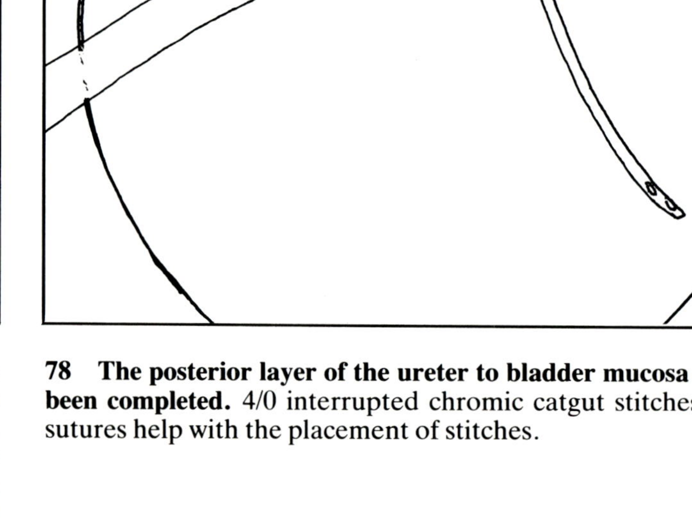

78   The posterior layer of the ureter to bladder mucosa anastomosis has been completed. 4/0 interrupted chromic catgut stitches are used. Stay sutures help with the placement of stitches.

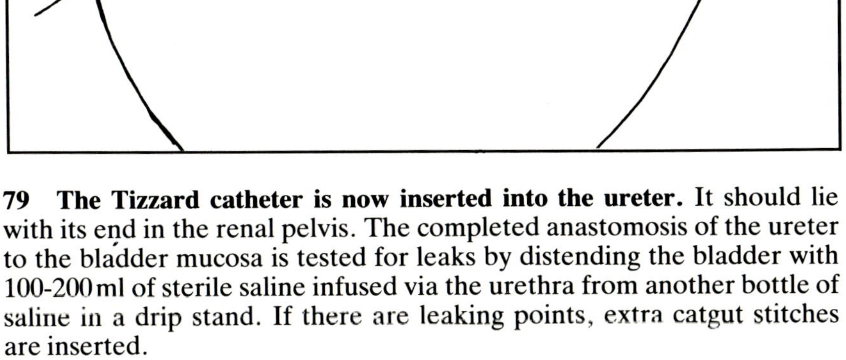

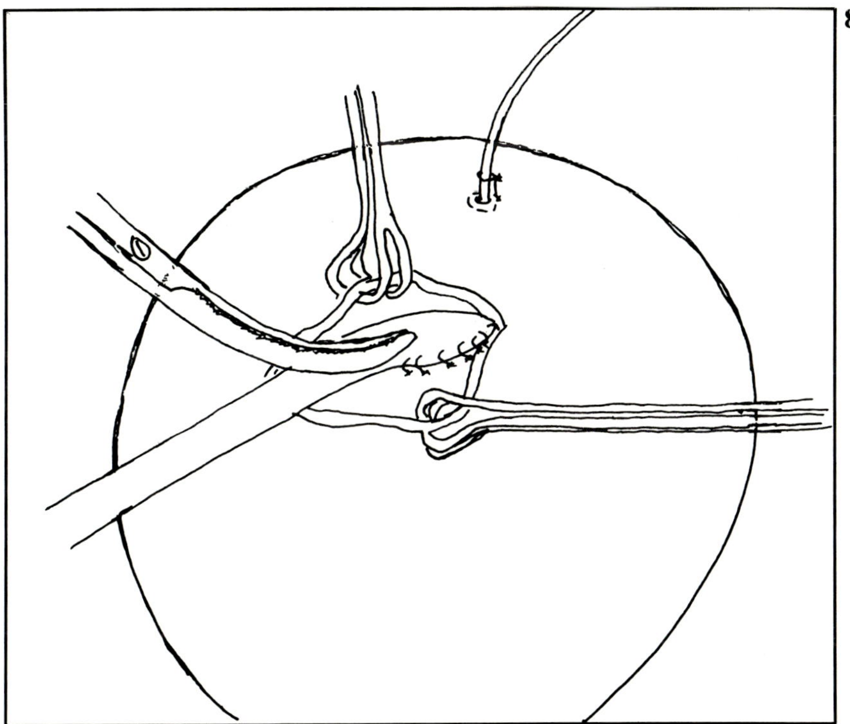

79 The Tizzard catheter is now inserted into the ureter. It should lie with its end in the renal pelvis. The completed anastomosis of the ureter to the bladder mucosa is tested for leaks by distending the bladder with 100-200 ml of sterile saline infused via the urethra from another bottle of saline in a drip stand. If there are leaking points, extra catgut stitches are inserted.

80 The muscle flaps have been grasped with Babcock forceps. The Tizzard catheter is shown emerging from the vault of the bladder. Moynihan forceps are placed on the distal ureter.

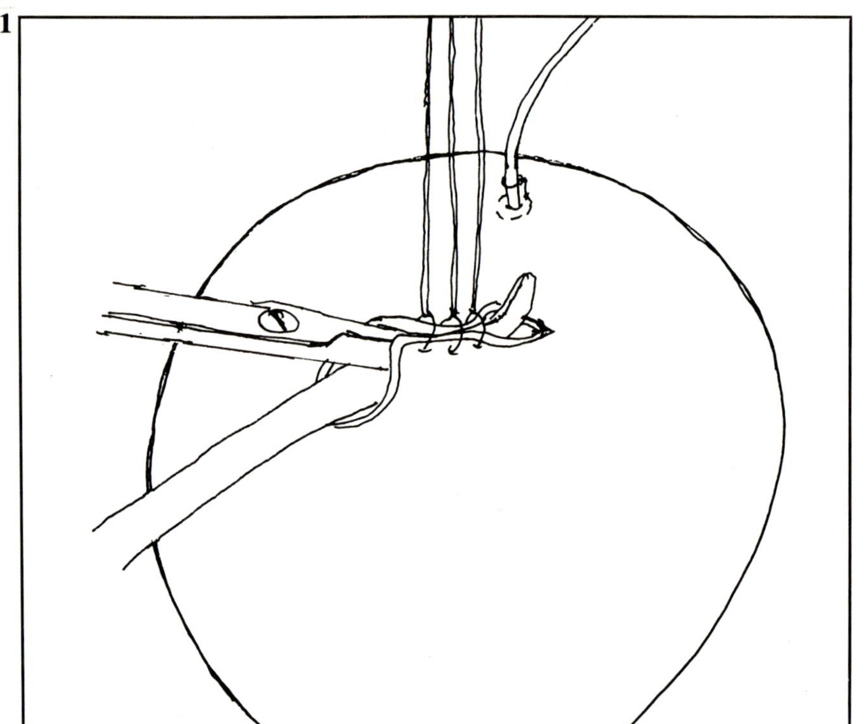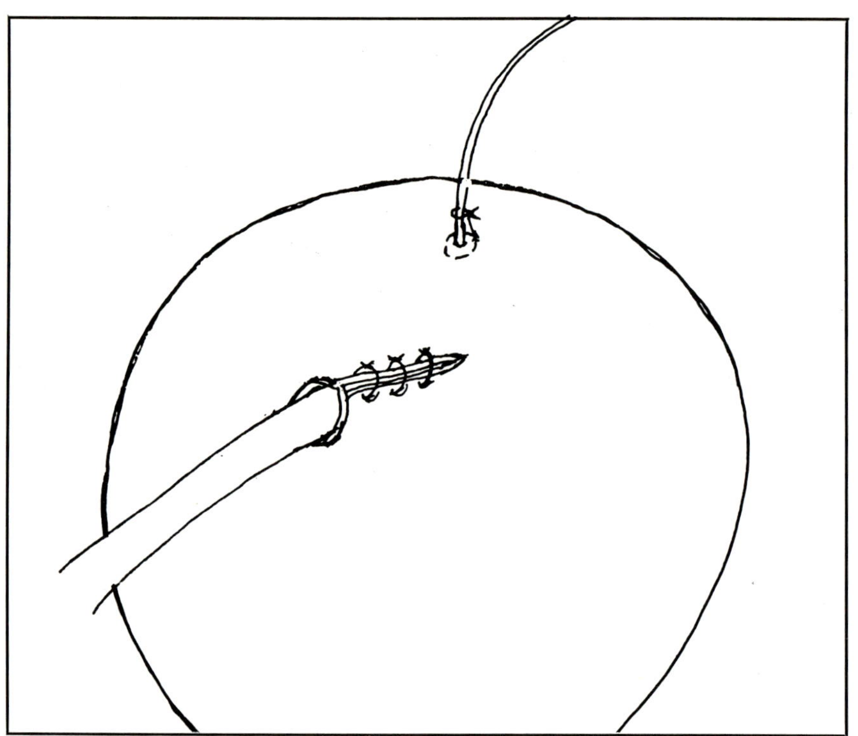

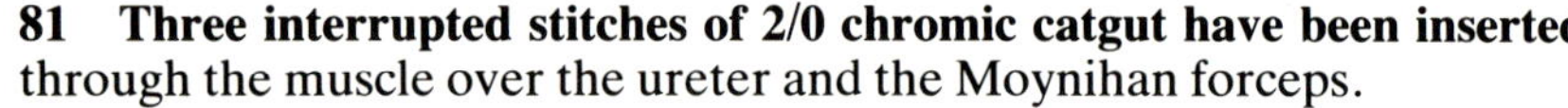

81 Three interrupted stitches of 2/0 chromic catgut have been inserted through the muscle over the ureter and the Moynihan forceps.

82 The Moynihan forceps is removed allowing snug, but not tight, fit of the ureter in the submucous tunnel.

83 Trimming of the ureter. The length of the ureter was too great for a comfortable lie. Therefore, the distal 4cm has been removed and the new end spatulated for anastomosis. The mucosa has a good pink colour.

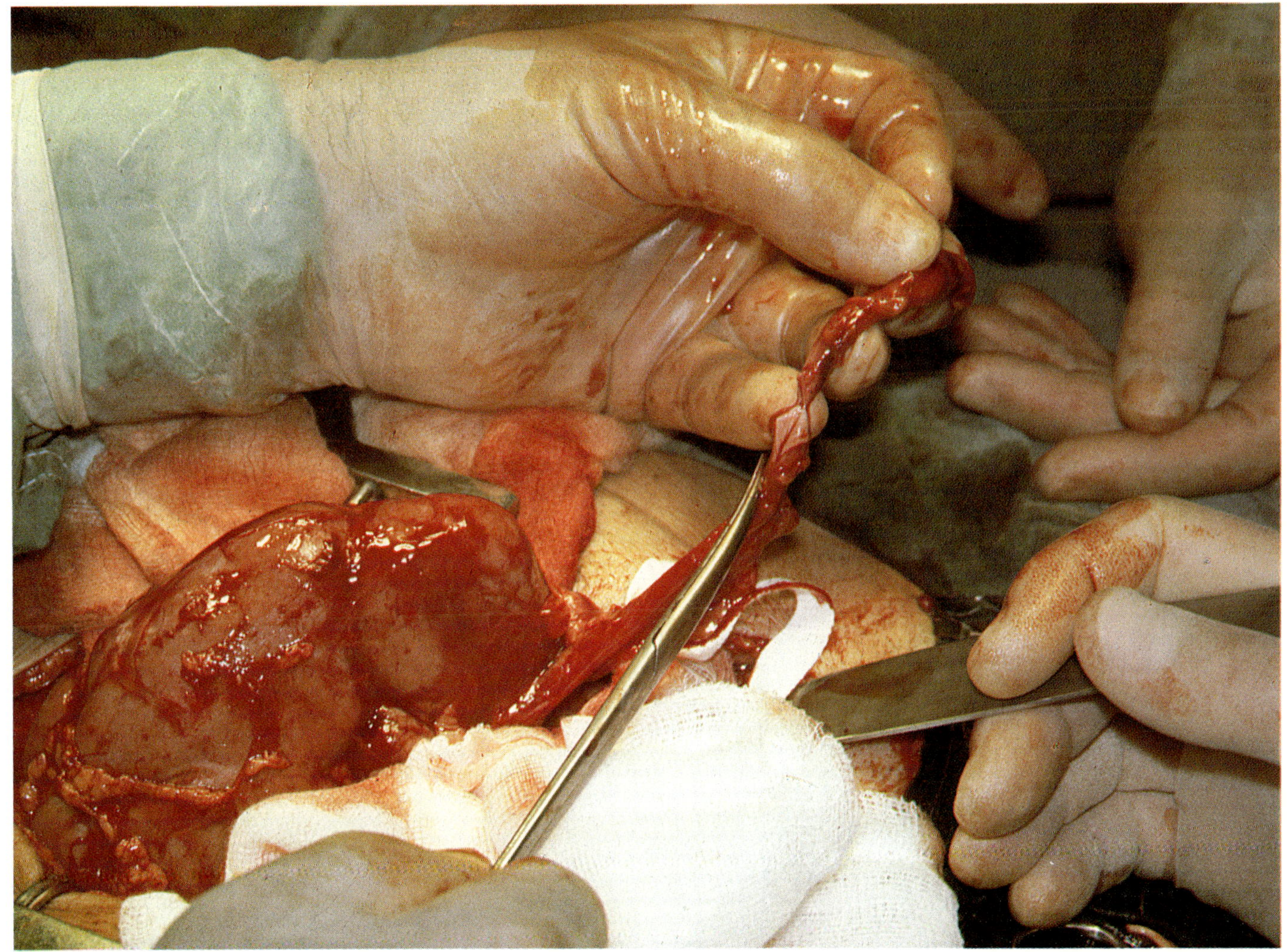

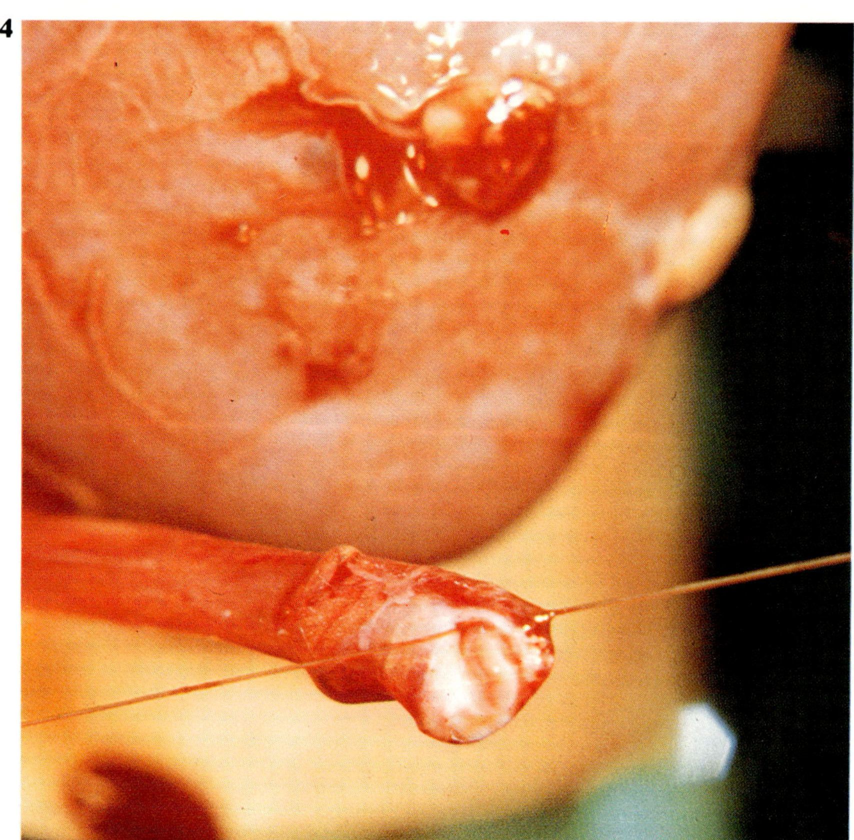

84 **Close-up view of spatulated end of ureter with first 4/0 catgut stitch inserted** near to the apex of the cut; the kidney is seen above.

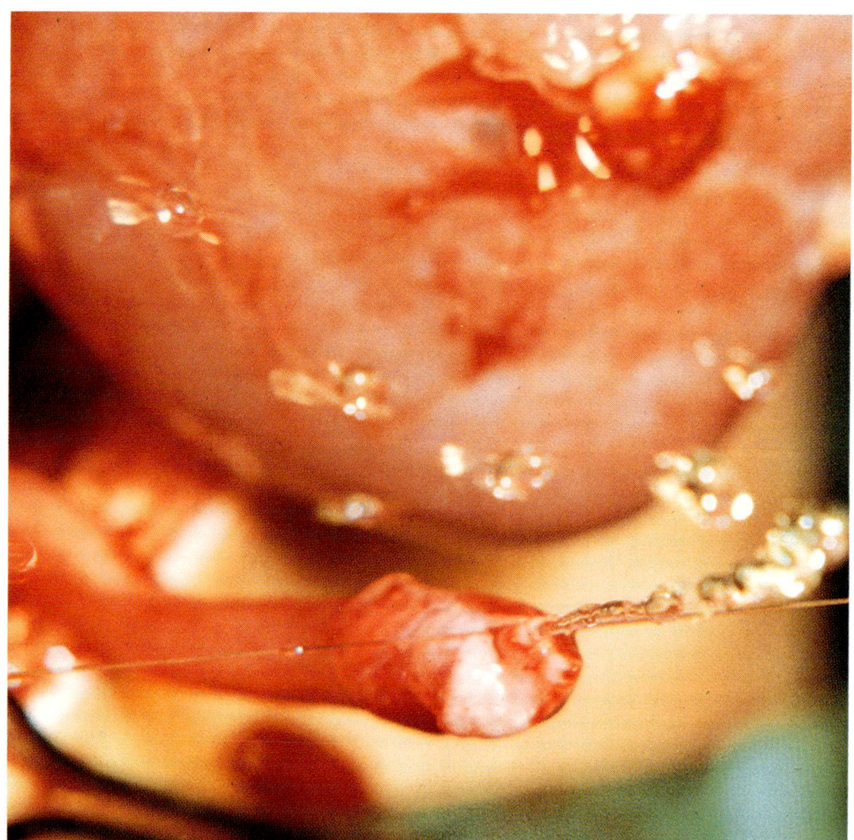

85 **Shows the first drops of urine being expelled by muscular contraction of the ureter.**

86 Dissection of the adventitial tissues over the bladder, which has been distended with 200 ml of saline via the urethral catheter. The muscle of the bladder has been incised allowing the mucosa to pout. The muscle is undermined so as to provide a tunnel after anastomosis of the ureter.

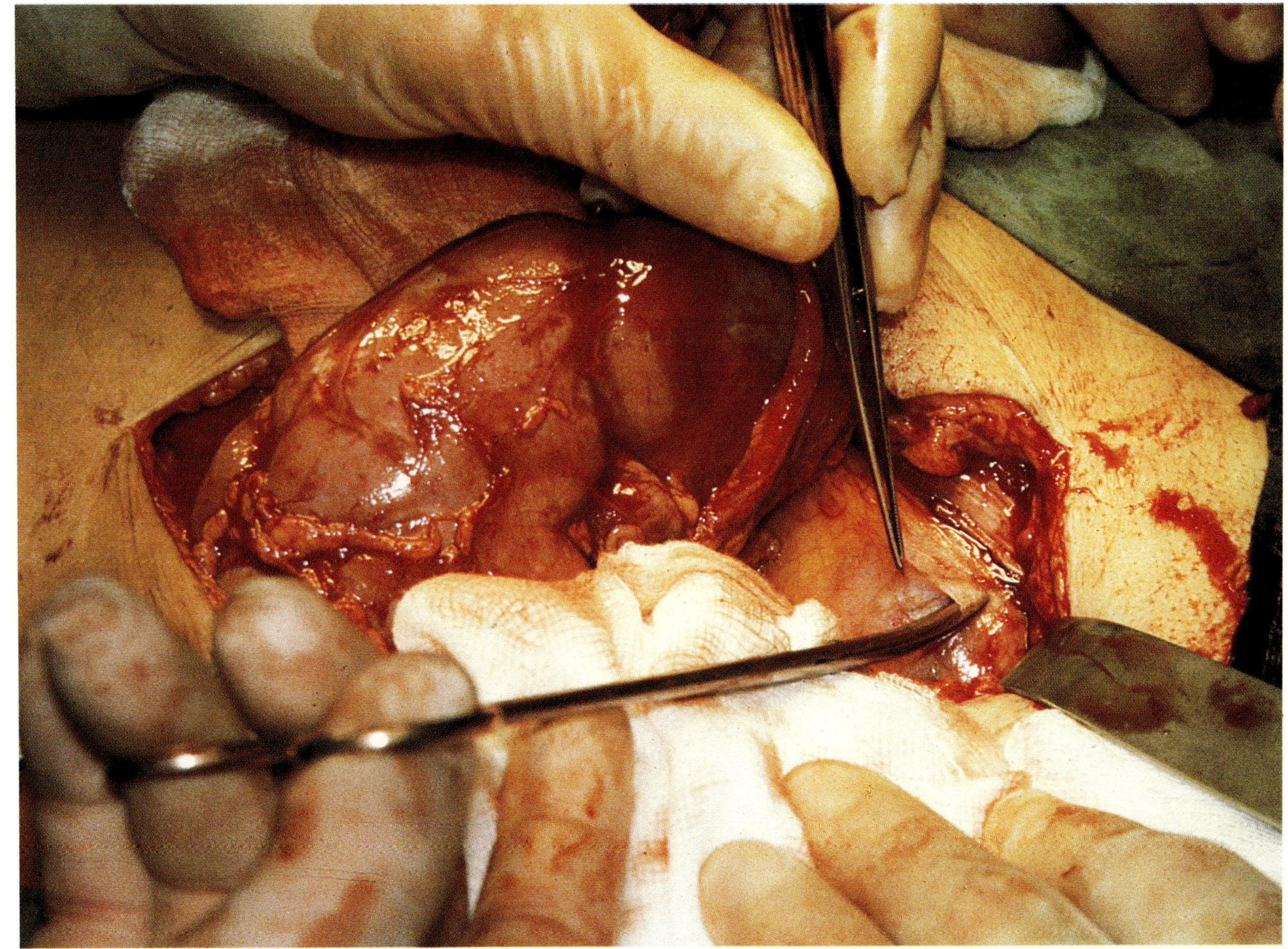

87 The dissection of the muscle in the submucus plane is completed.

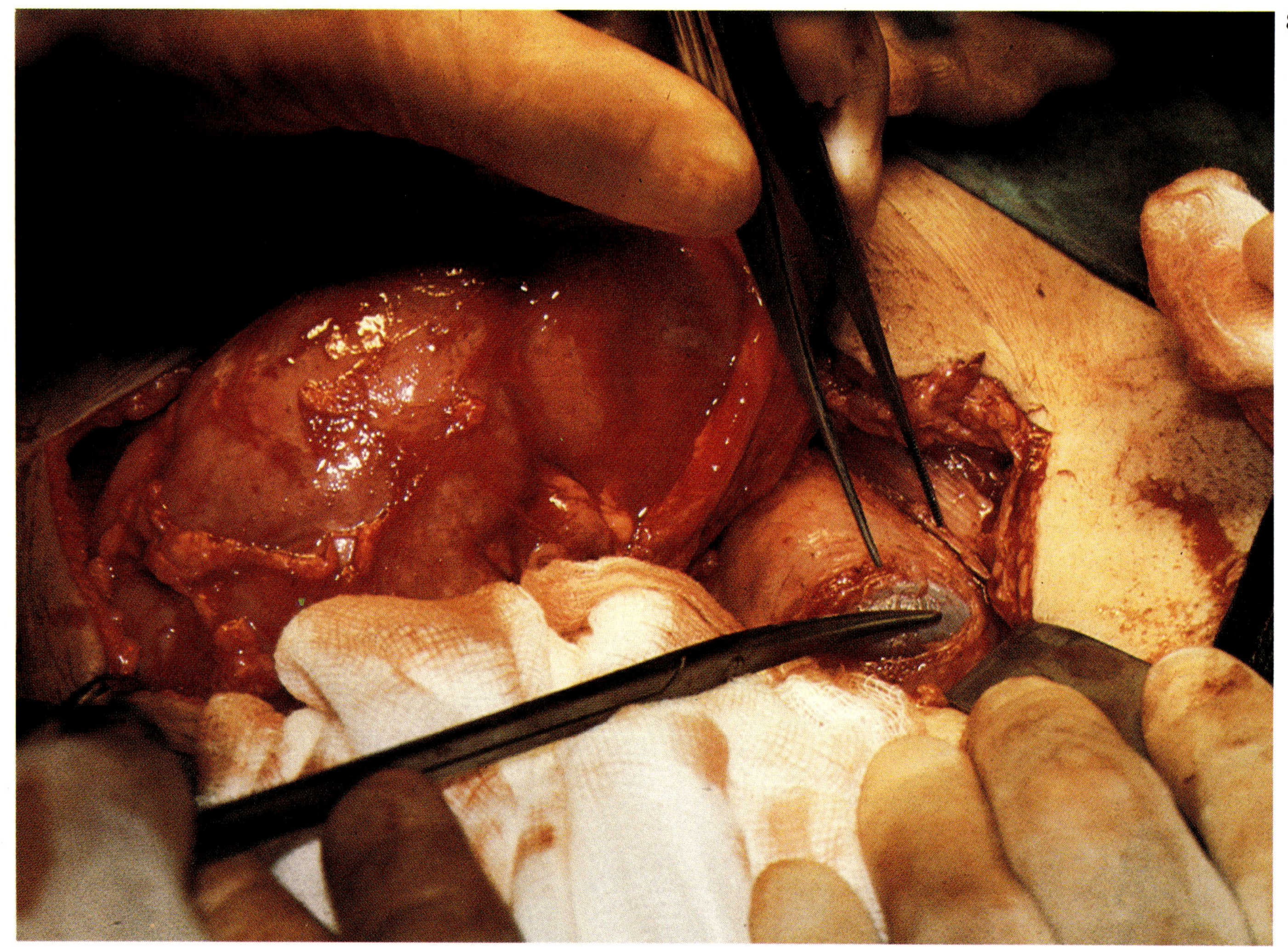

88 The bladder muscle has been stripped back to form flaps that will be sewn over the ureter. The muscle is held in Babcock forceps on each side.

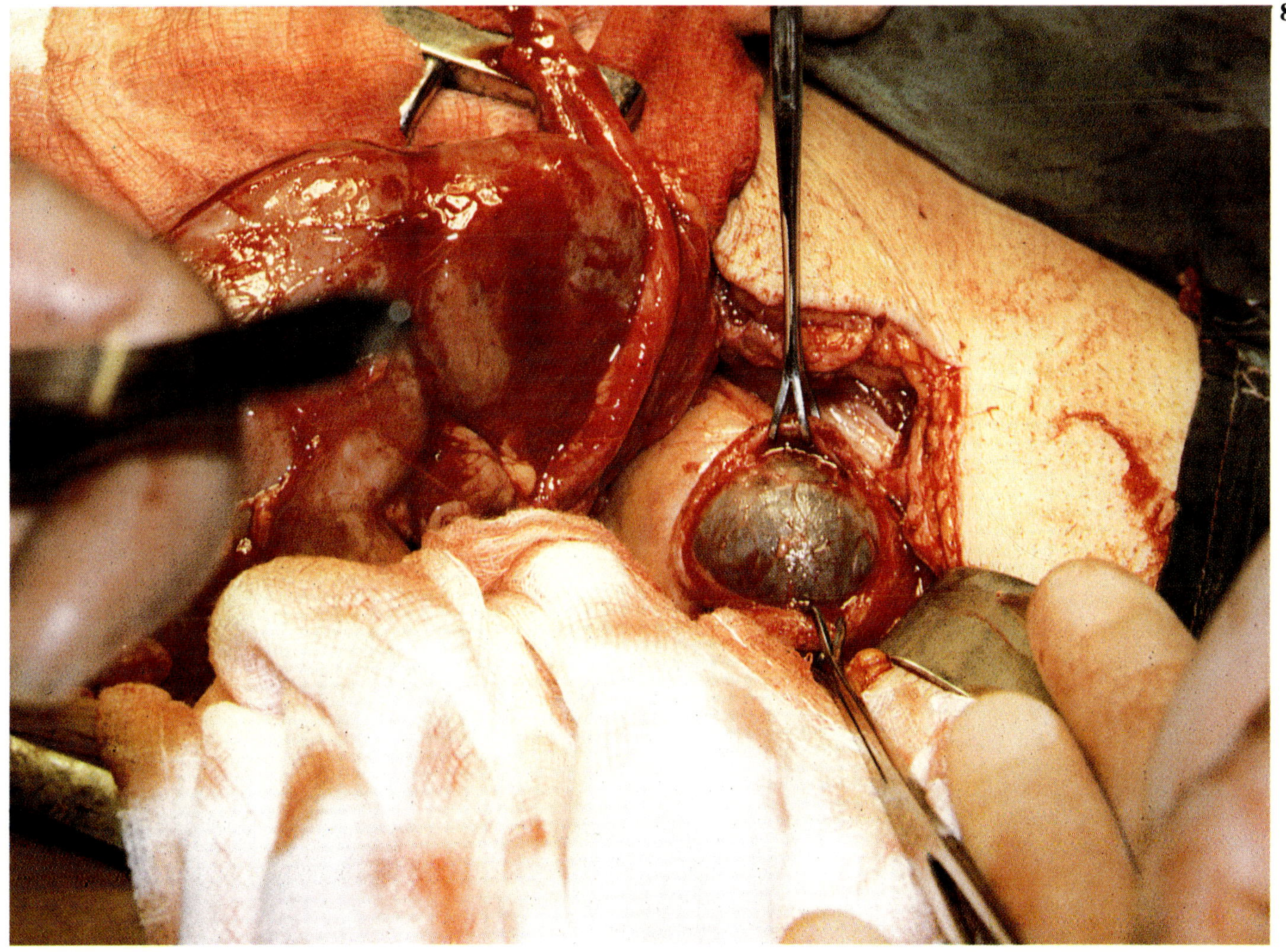

89 Incision into the bladder at the distal inferior extremity of the dissection. Sterile saline infused into the bladder is escaping and is aspirated.

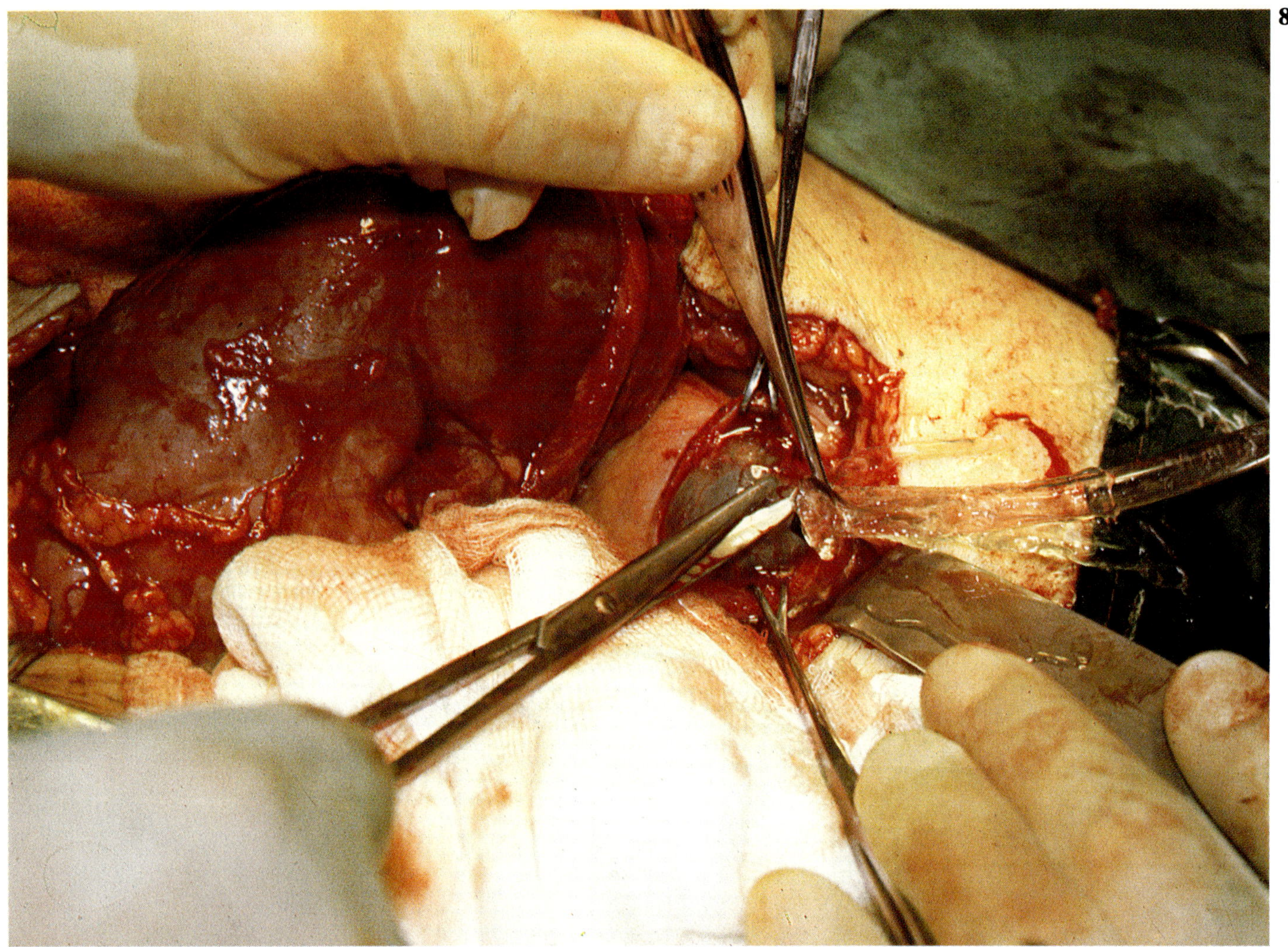

90   A right angle forceps has been passed through the cystotomy to a point some 2 cm medial, where the further incision is made over the tip of the right angle forceps. A No. 6 Tizzard catheter will be drawn through this incision.

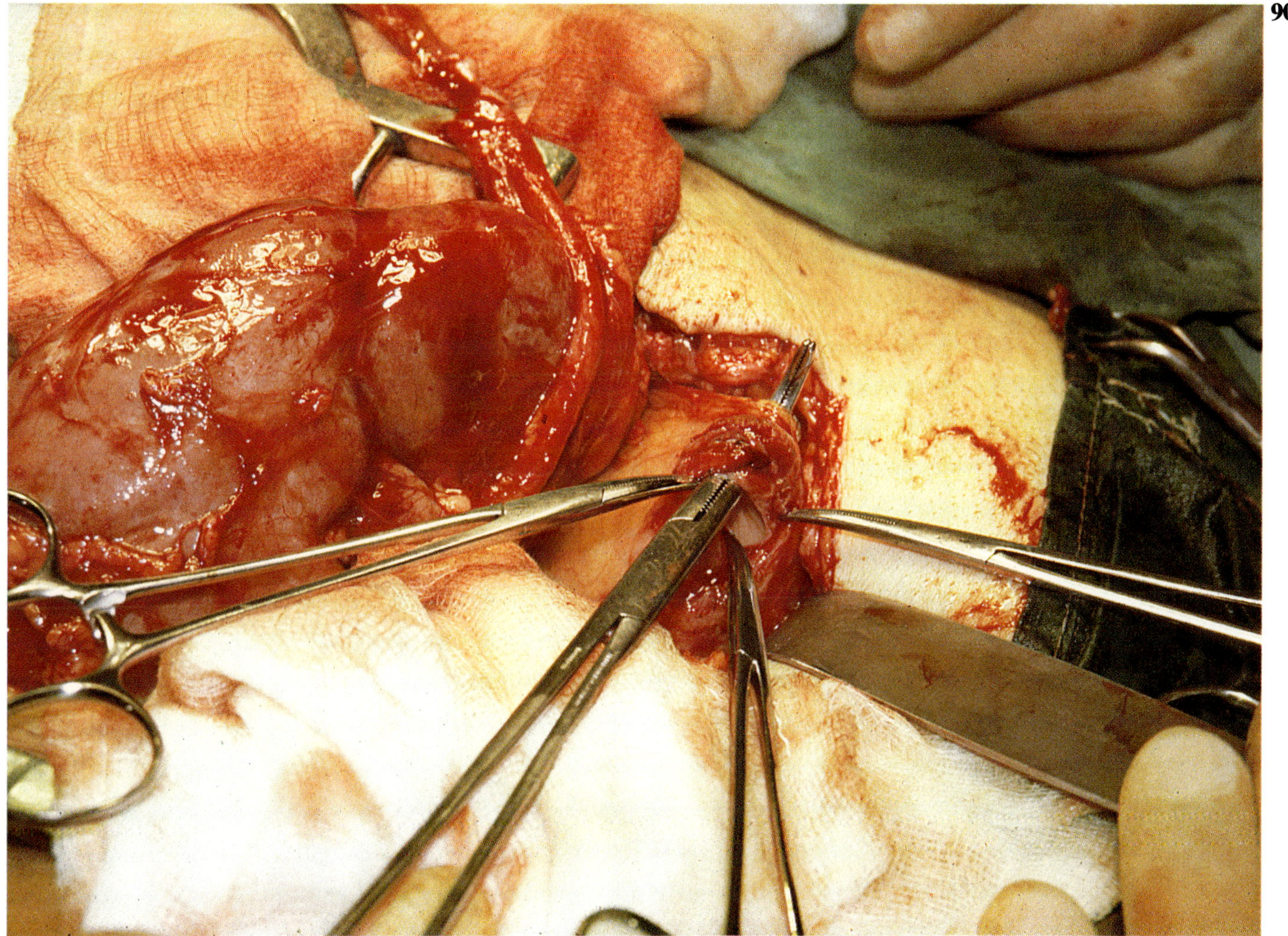

91   The Tizzard catheter grasped by the right angle forceps.

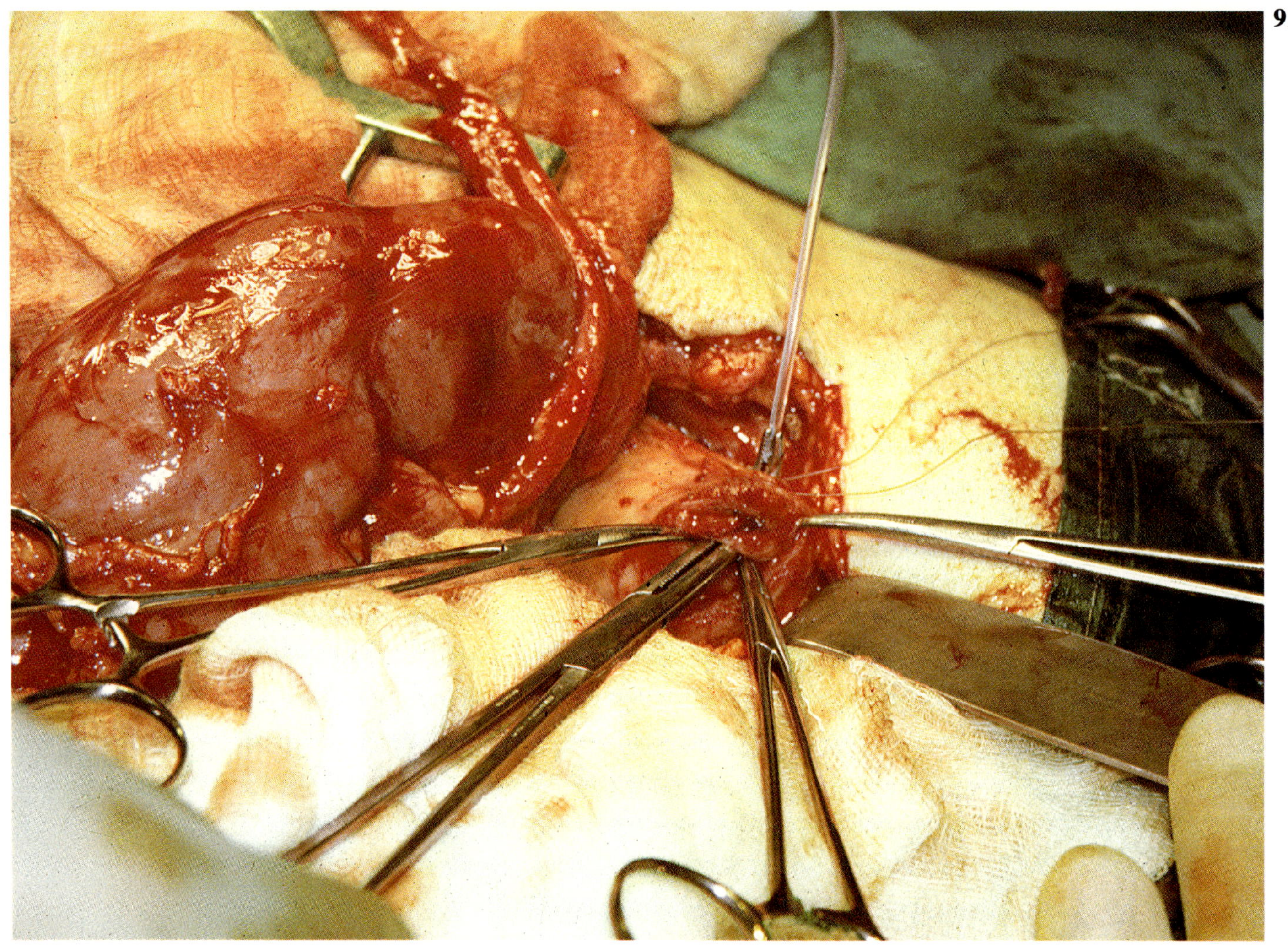

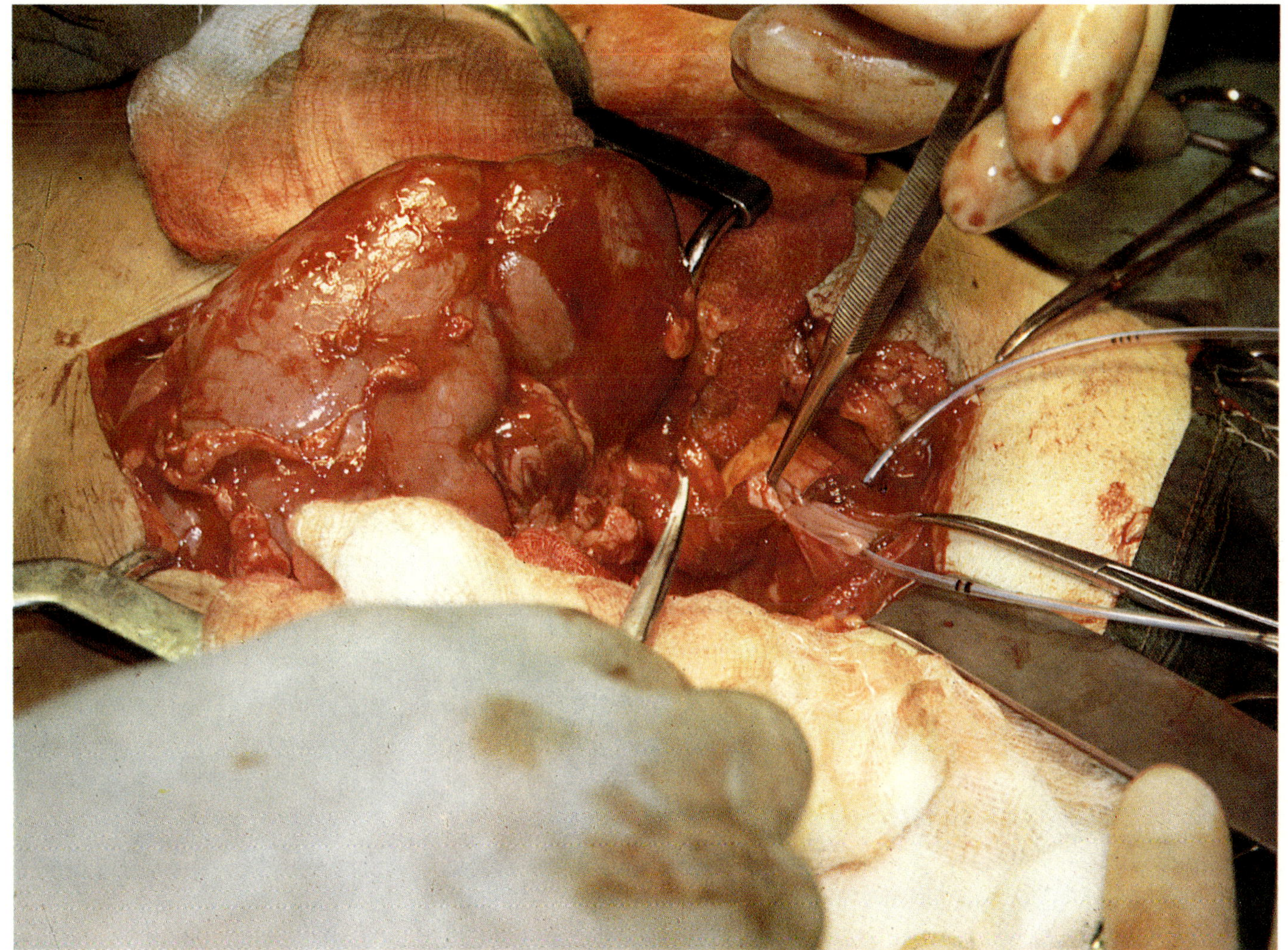

92 **The Tizzard catheter brought out through the cystotomy.** A 2/0 catgut purse-string suture through the bladder wall encircles the emerging catheter.

93

93 Several interrupted catgut stitches have been placed through the full thickness of the ureter and the mucosa of the bladder. The Tizzard catheter has been passed up the lumen of the ureter.

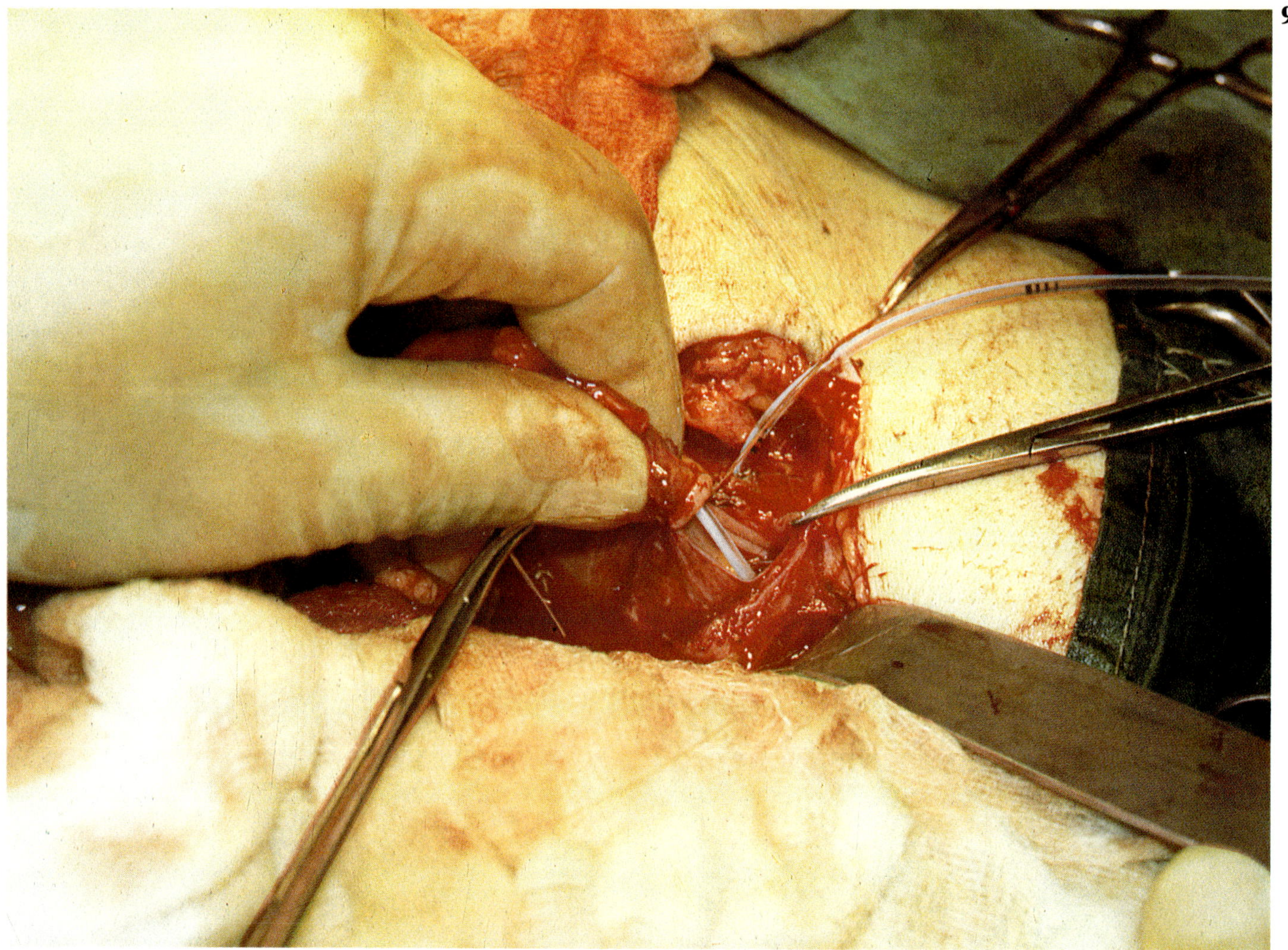

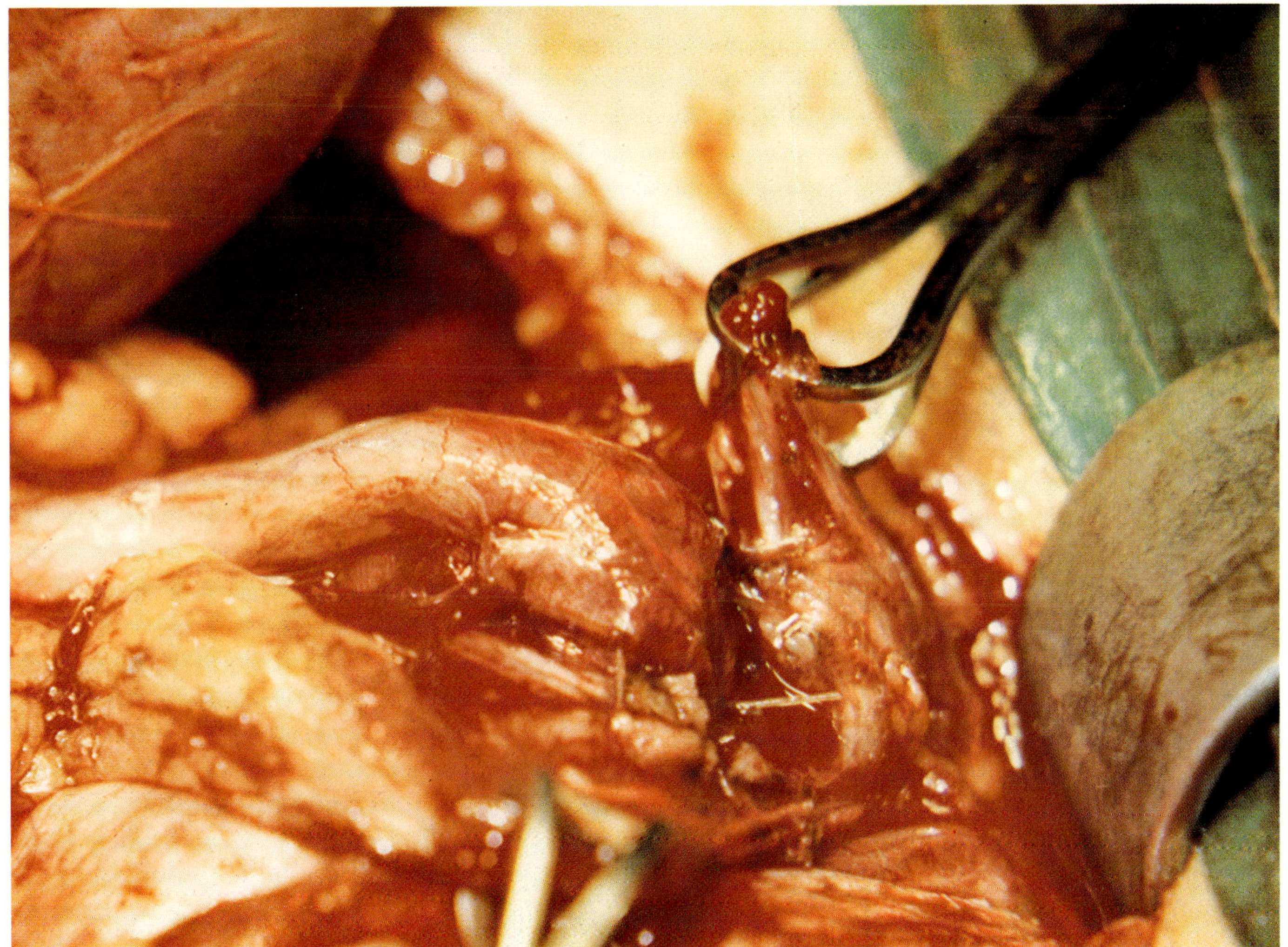

94 Close-up to show bladder muscle being elevated in preparation for construction of anti-reflux submucous tunnel.

95 A further 200 ml of saline have been infused into the bladder through the urethral catheter, to define any leaks. A Moynihan forceps has been laid over the terminal ureter so as to ensure that the tunnel, when it is constructed, will not be too tight. The first 2/0 chromic catgut stitch has been inserted through the muscle on each side of the ureter.

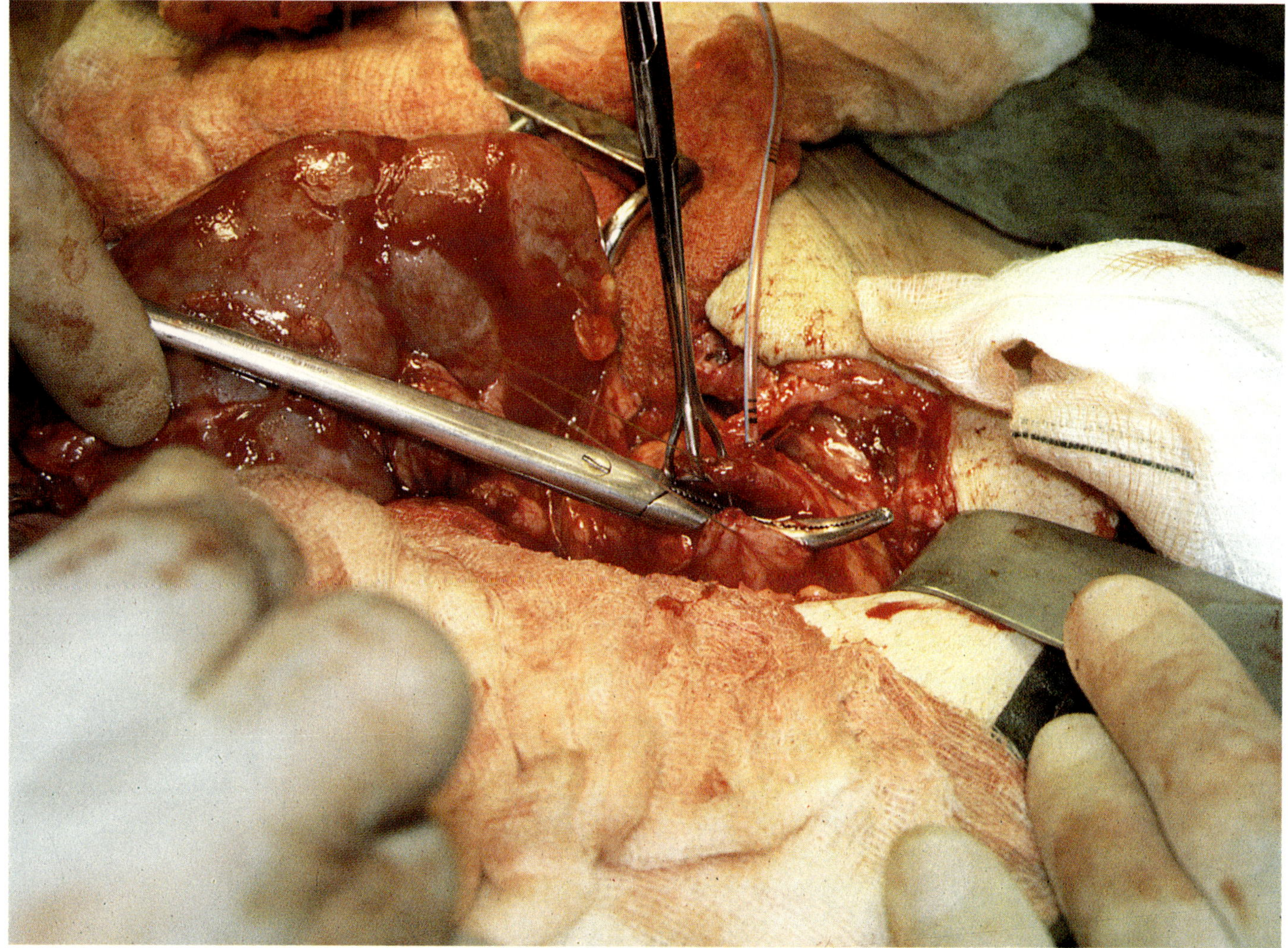

96   Close-up to show how the Moynihan forceps protect the ureter from being constricted when the muscular tunnel is constructed.

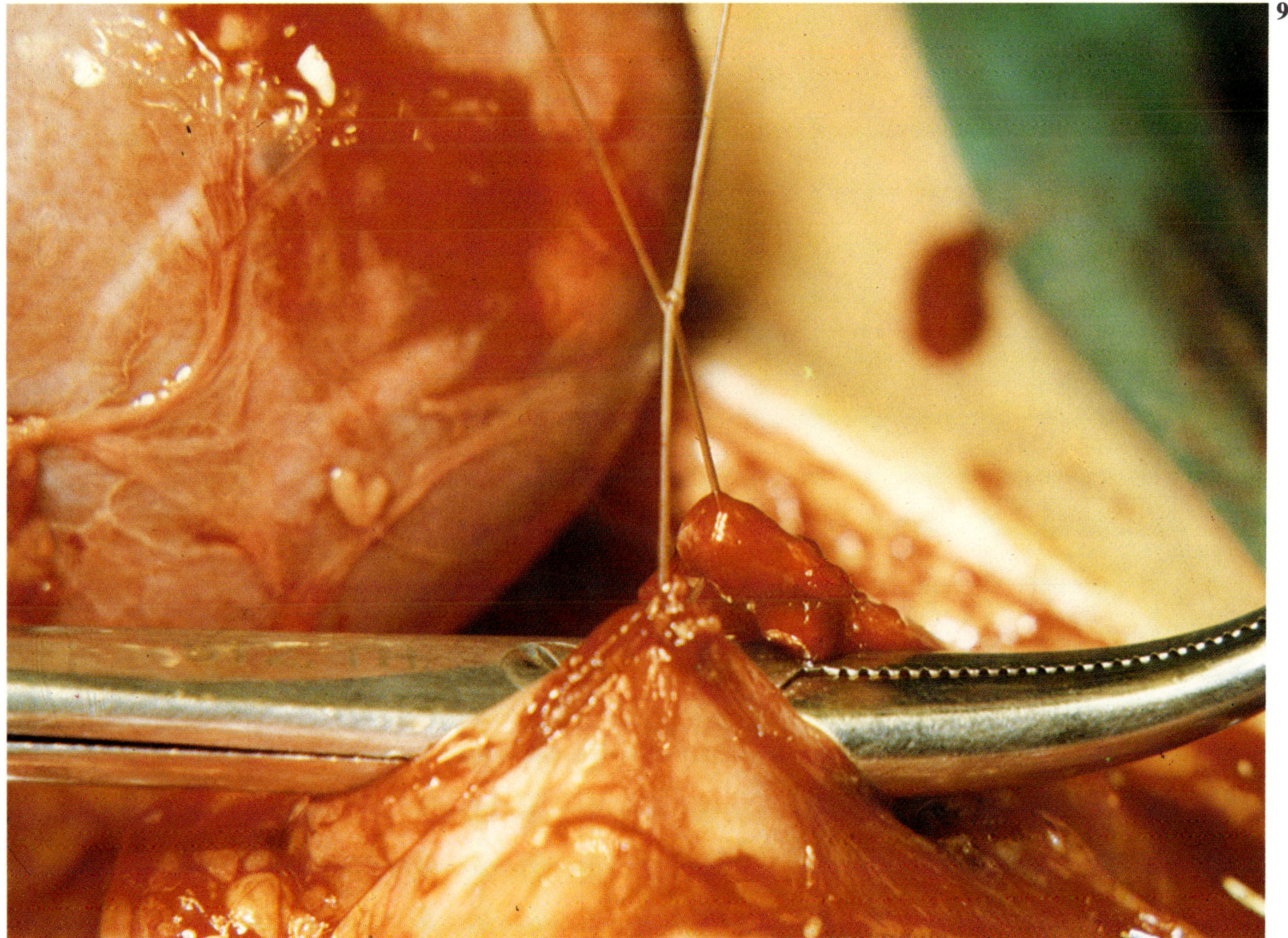

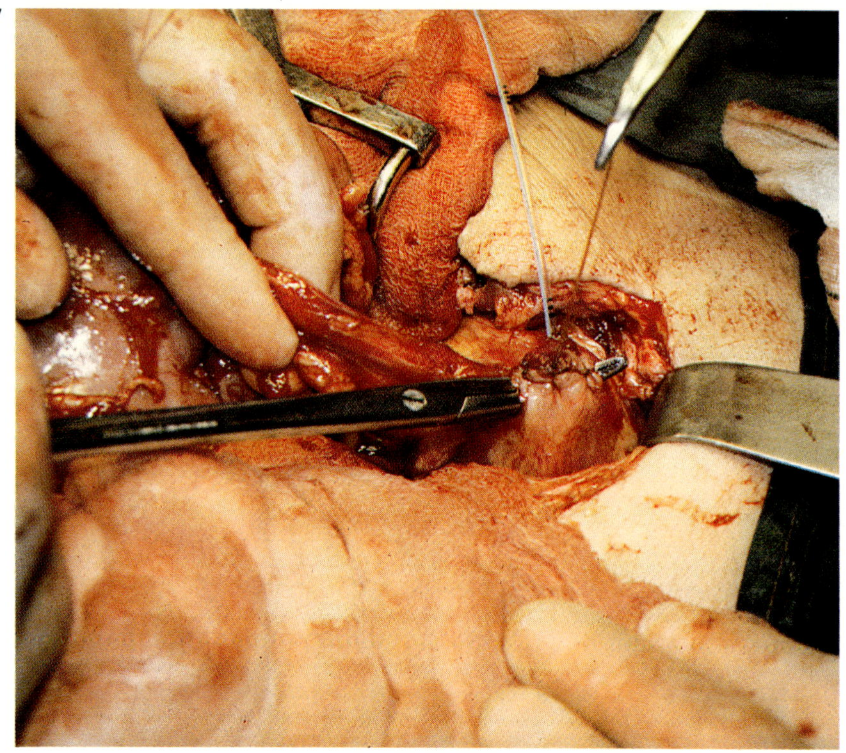

97 **The tunnel has now been completed with three catgut stitches.** The Moynihan forceps demonstrates that the tunnel is loose enough to avoid constriction of the terminal ureter.

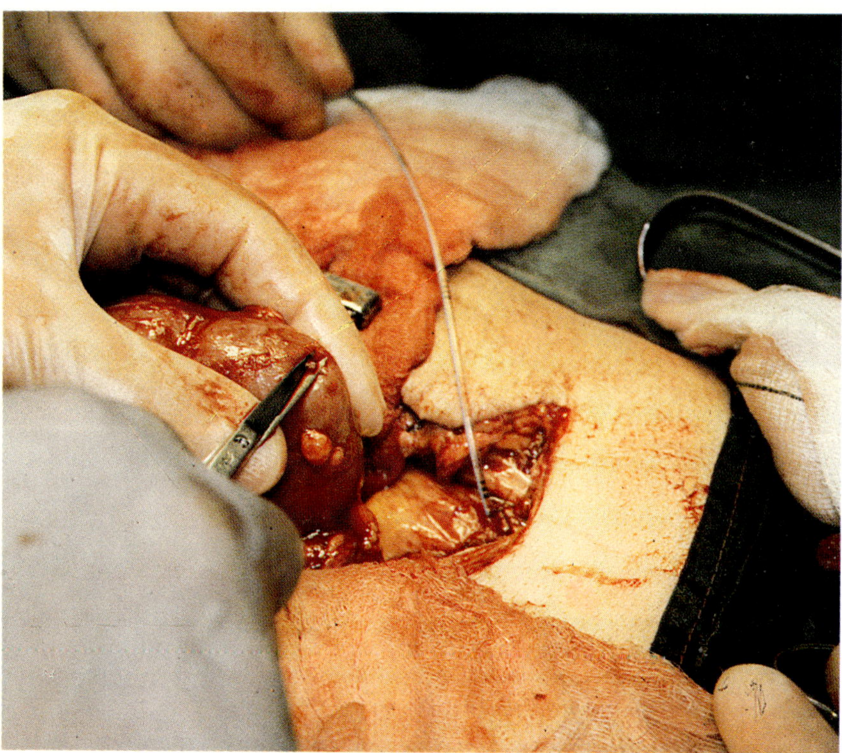

98 **A small biopsy has been taken from the surface of the lower pole of the kidney.**

99 The kidney has taken up a 'comfortable' position in the extraperitoneal plane of the right iliac fossa. A large tube drain has been brought out through the upper extremity of the wound. This is left in until it stops draining, usually on the second or third day. The capsulotomy can be seen and the Tizzard catheter is emerging to the right through a stab incision some 3cm from the wound extremity.

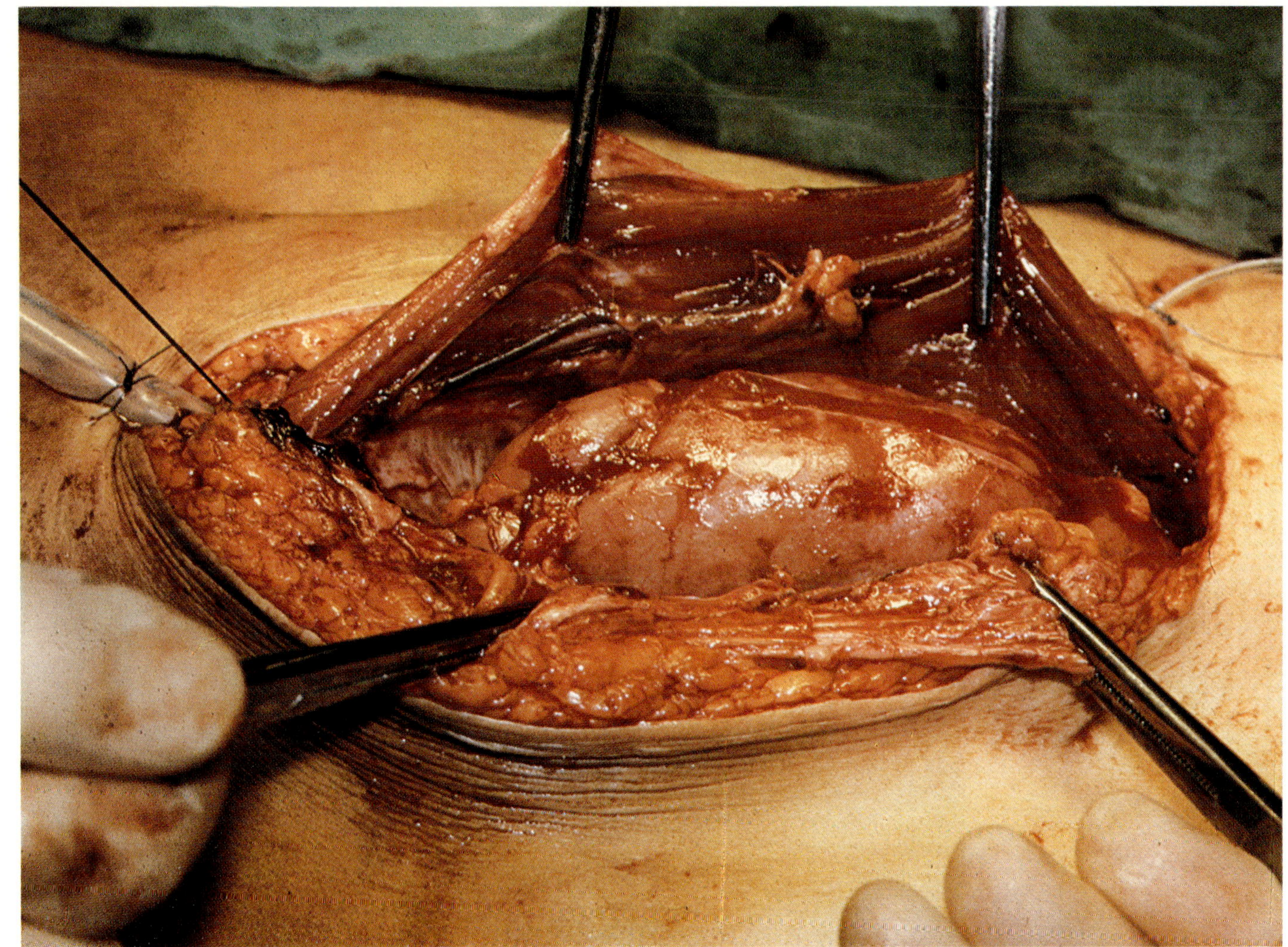

100 The wound has been closed. The drainage tube and the Tizzard catheter can be seen clearly. Urine is coming out of the Tizzard catheter.

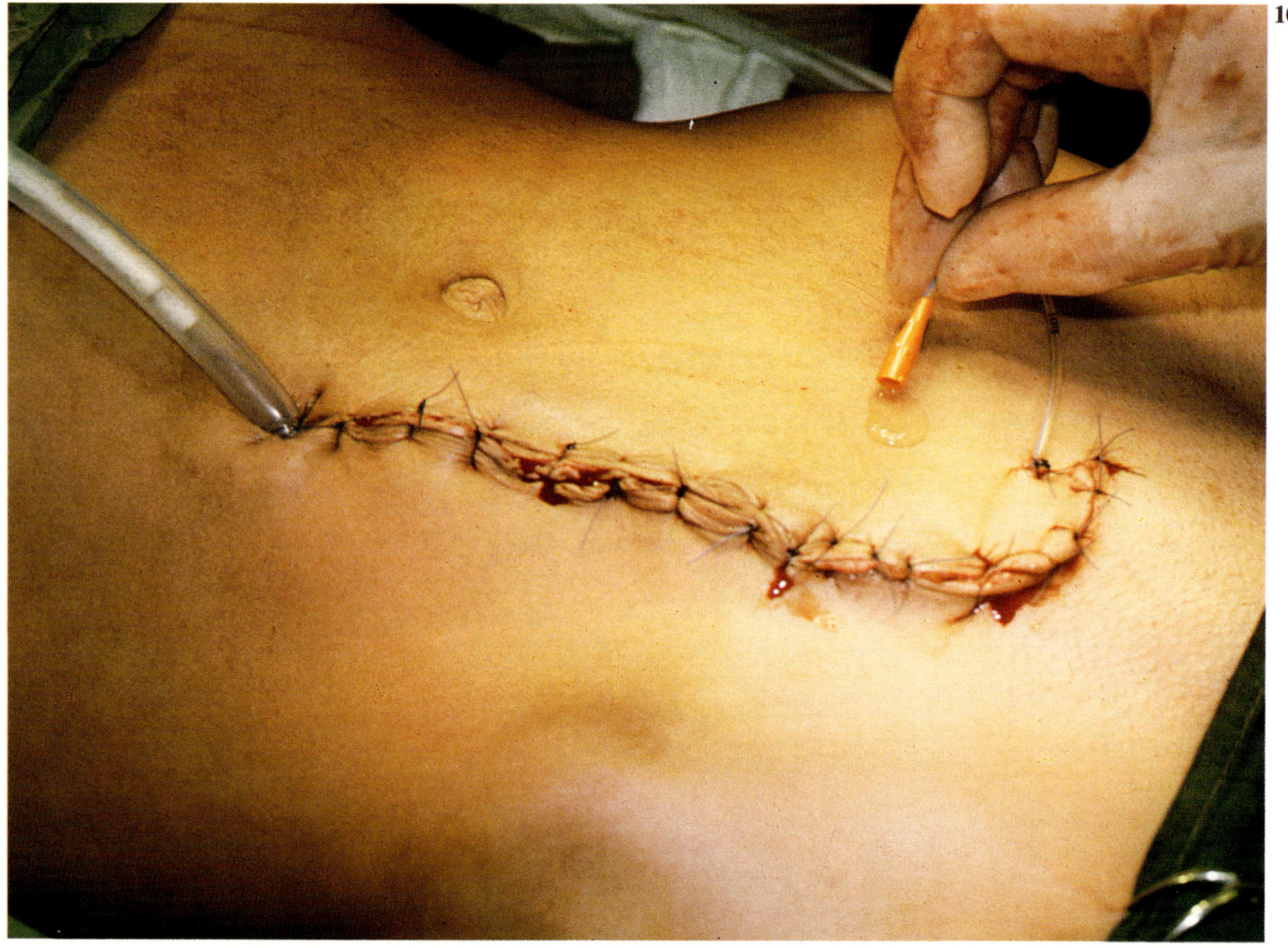

Alternative method of transplantation of an adult kidney in a child

101   Midline lower
abdominal incision.

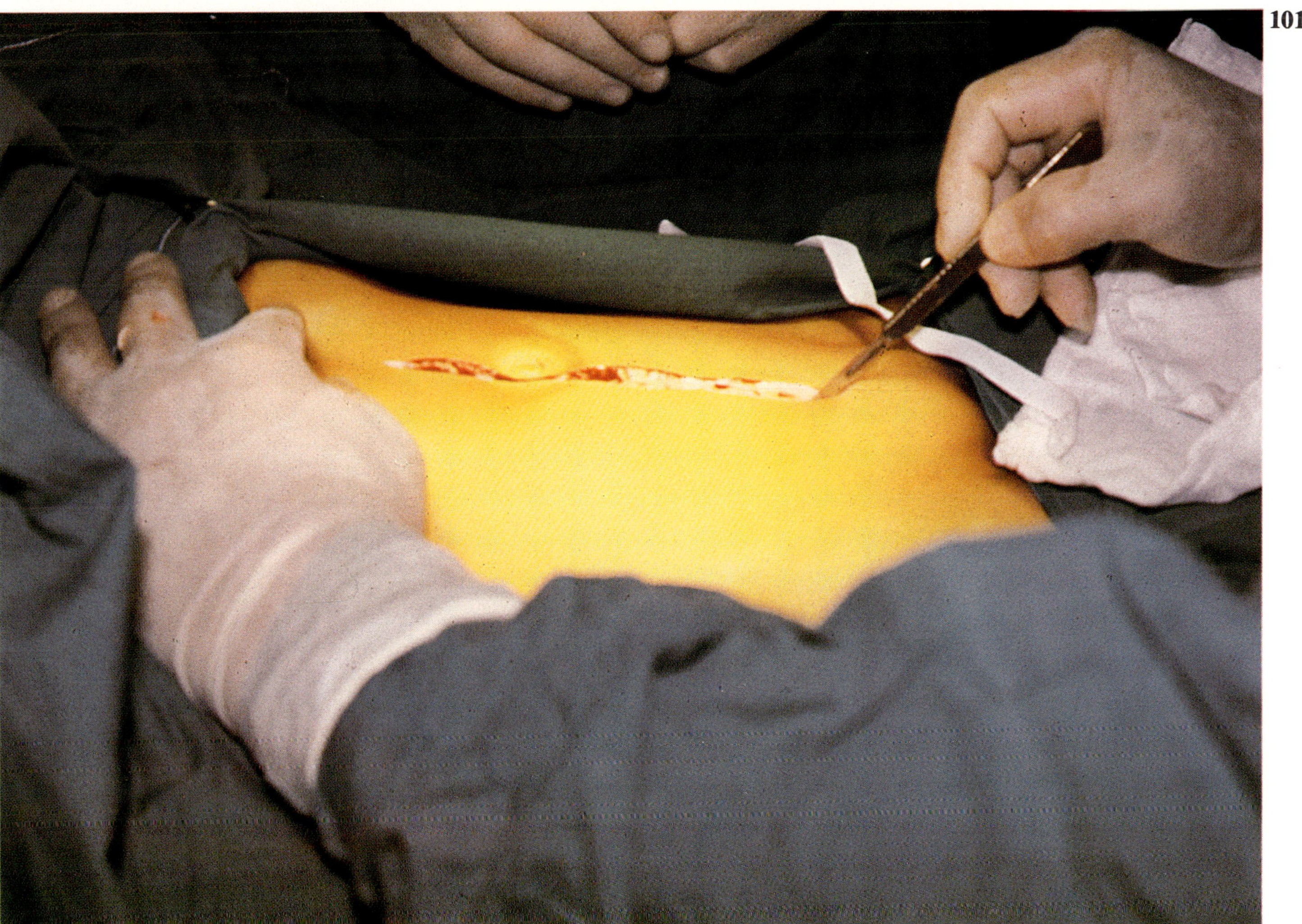

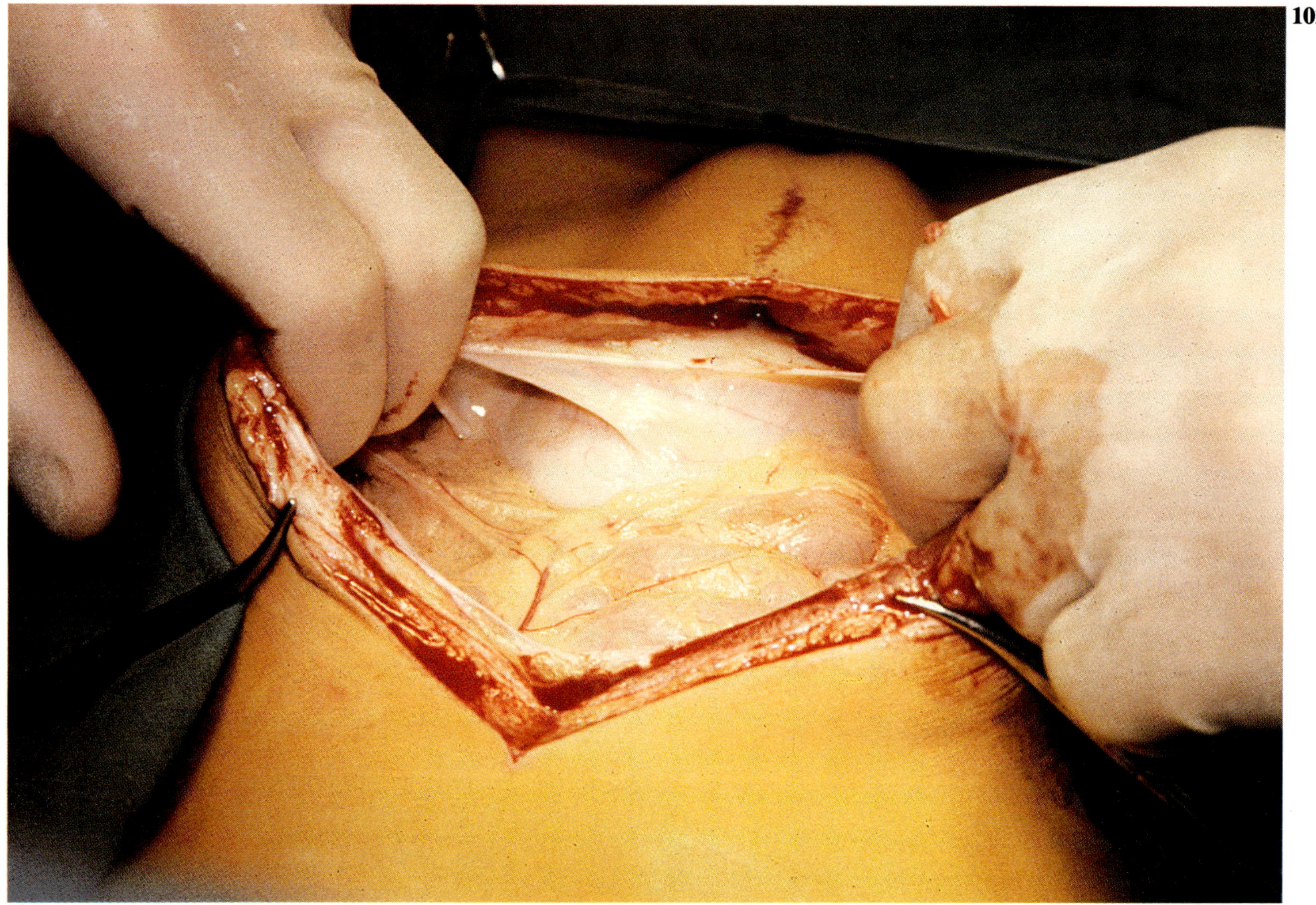

103

103 Exposure and control of right common iliac artery above and vein below. Bifurcation of the common iliac artery shown to the left.

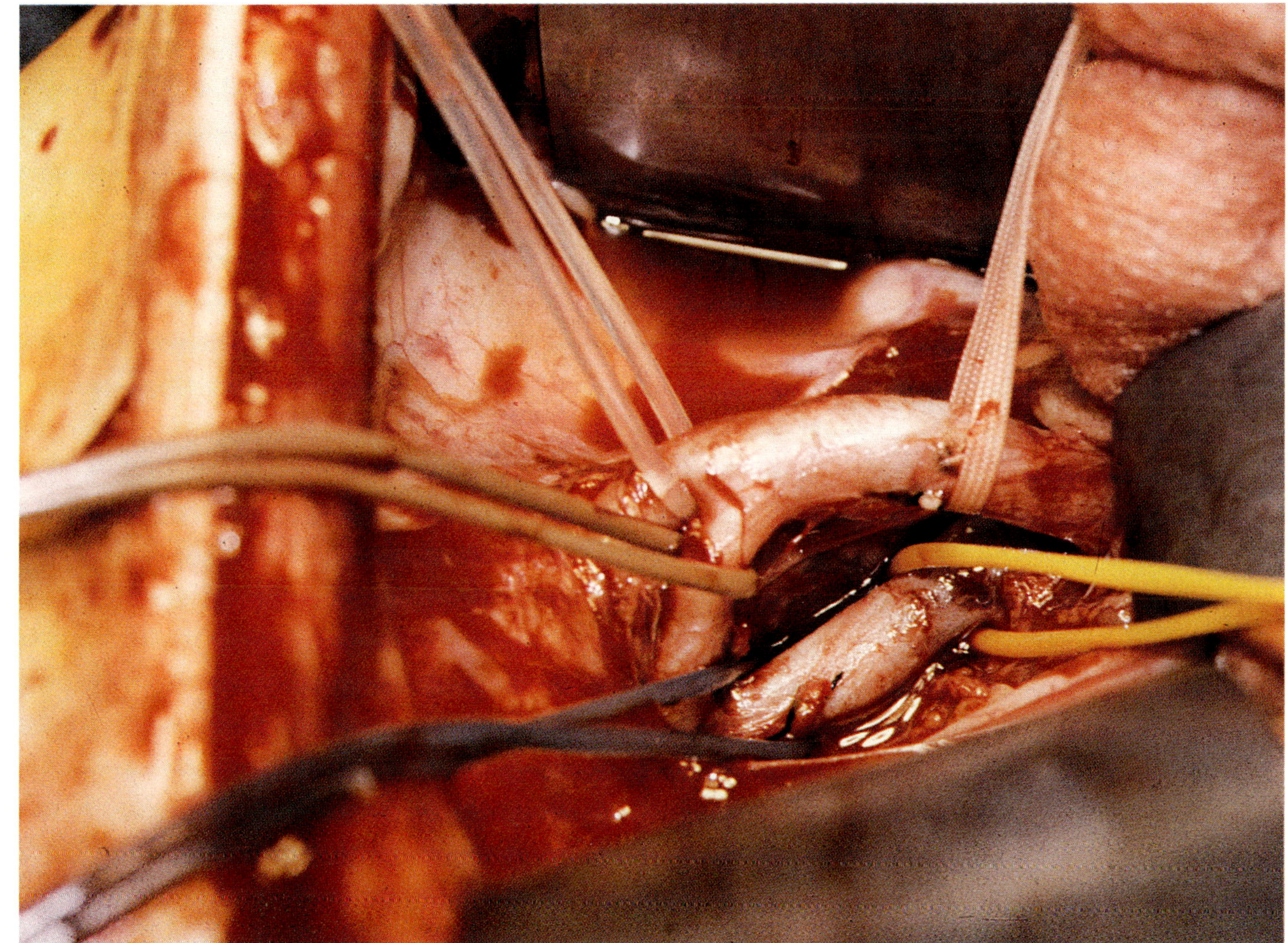

104 The vein has been clamped with two bulldog clips, an anterior incision has been made in the vein, and the first 5/0 prolene stitch has been passed through the proximal extremity.

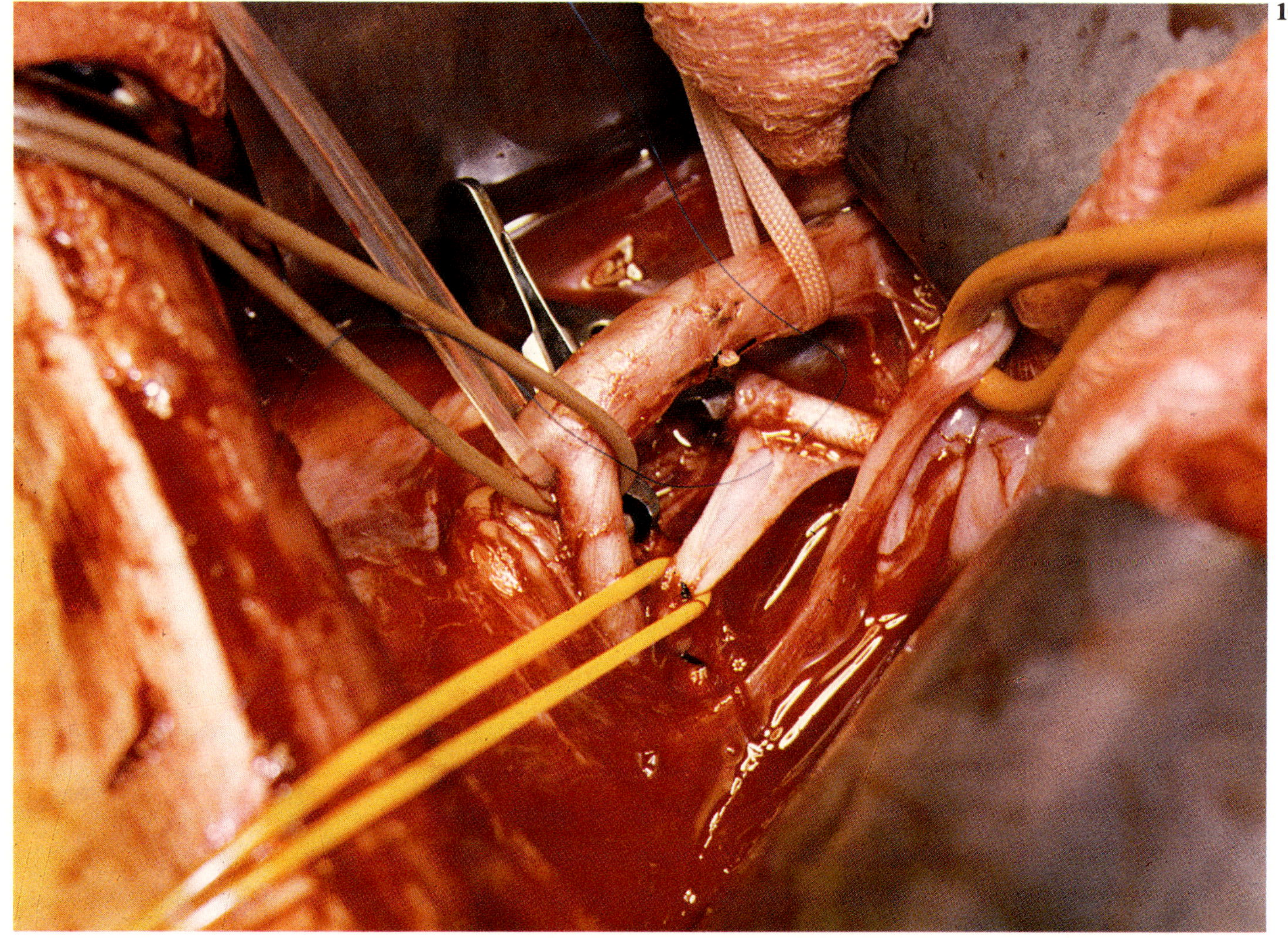

105 Venous anastomosis posterior wall completed from within.

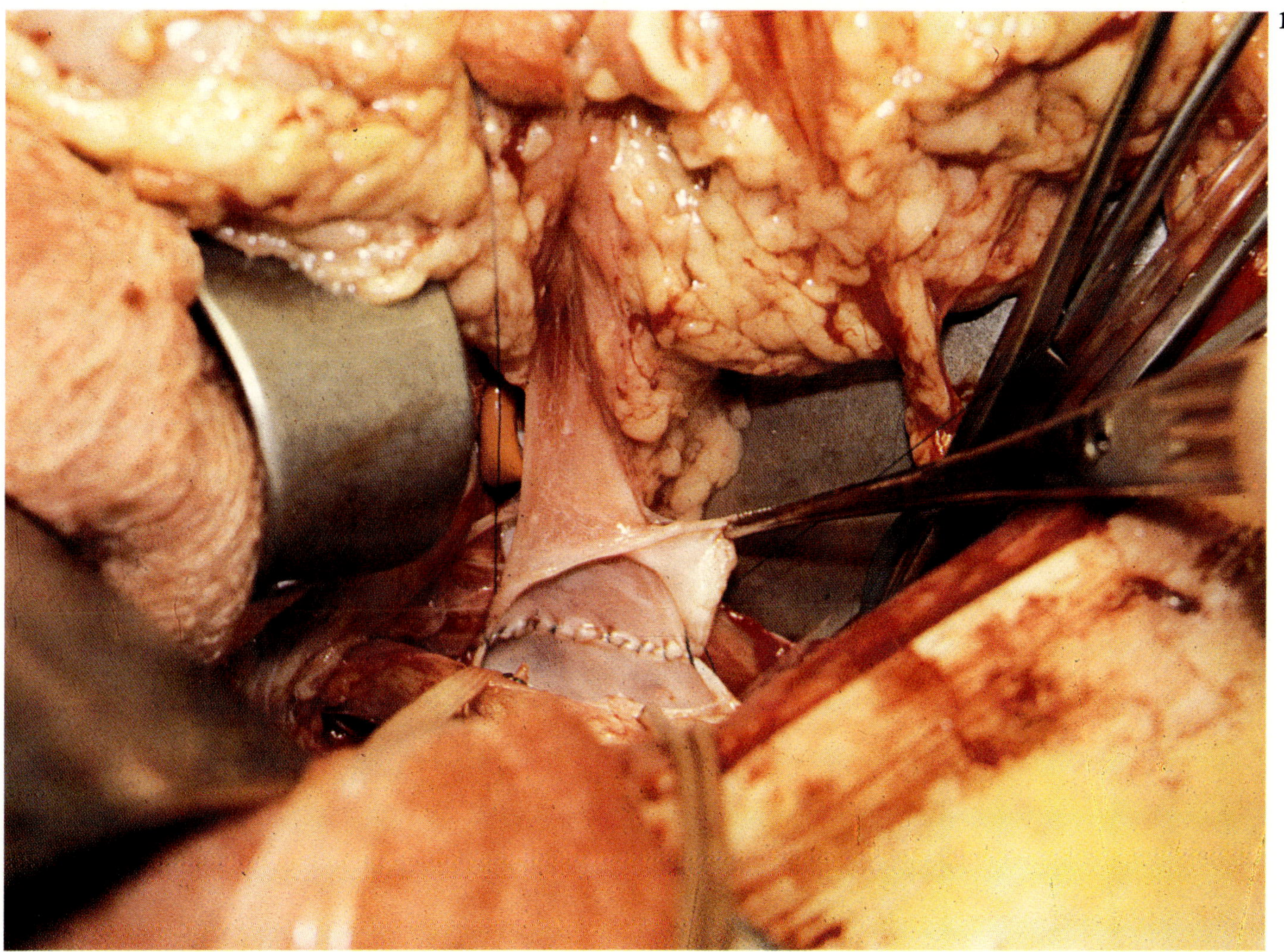

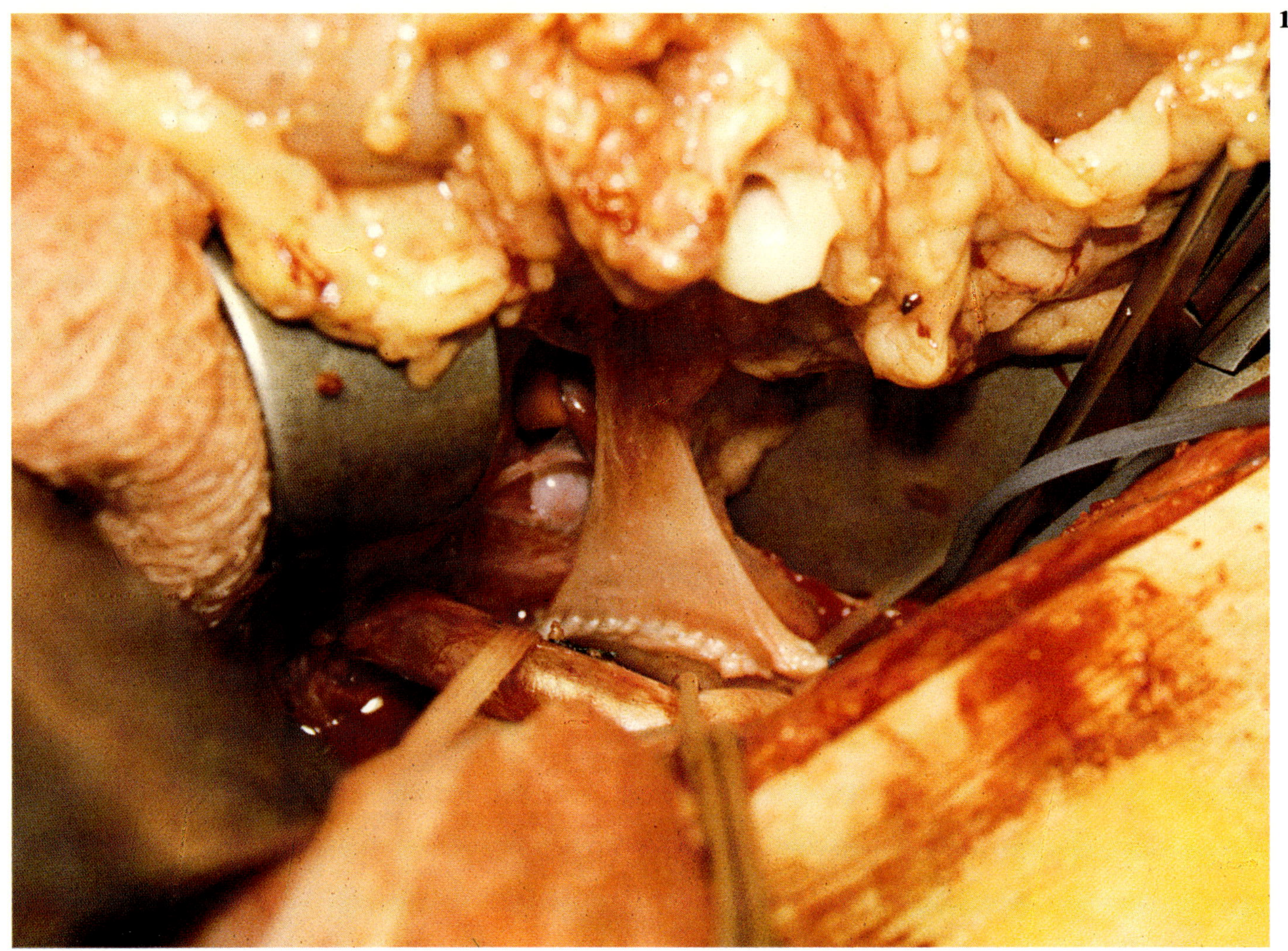

107 The common iliac artery has been clamped and an anterior incision has been made with Potts scissors.

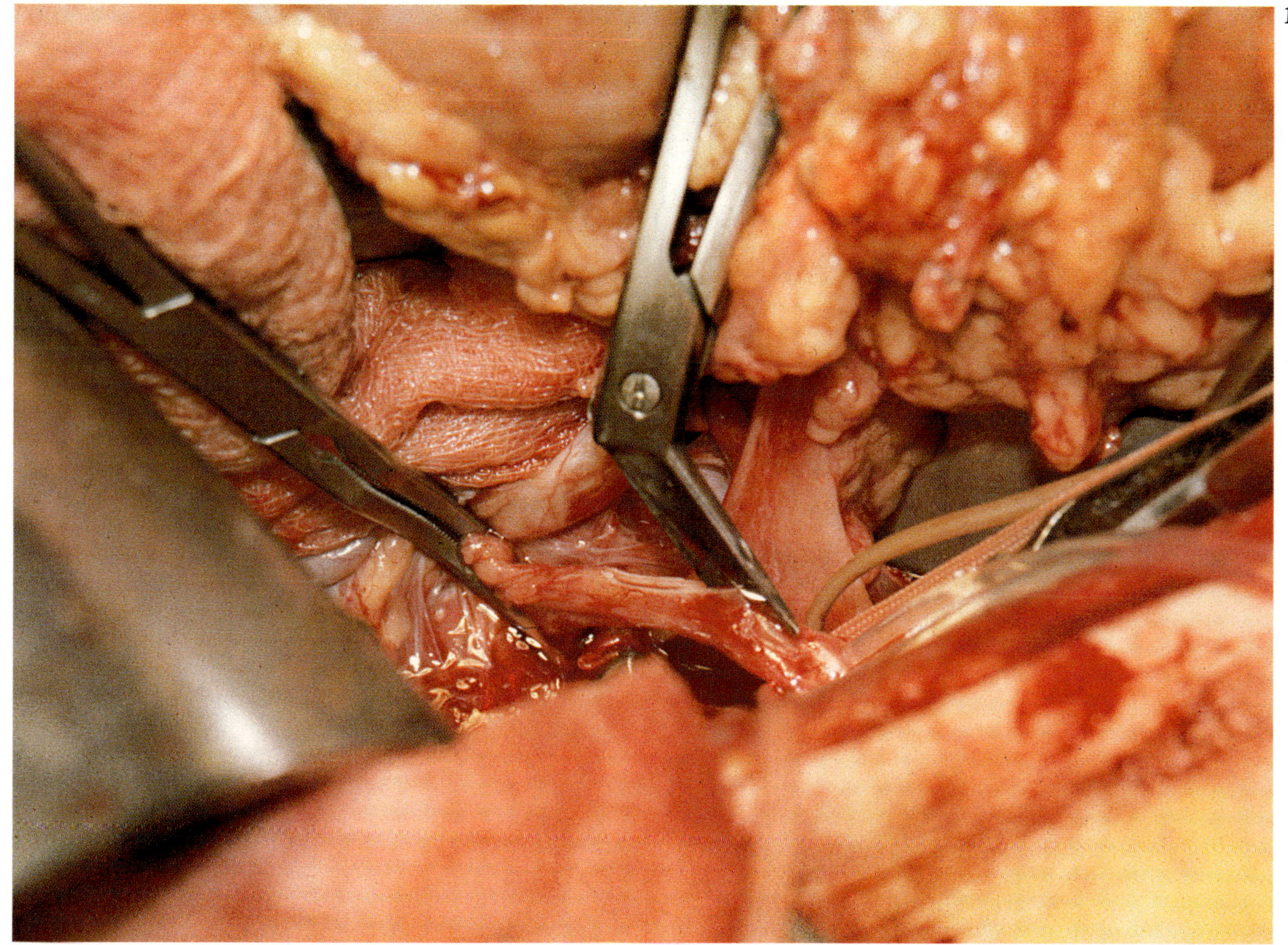

108 The kidney is not yet perfused. The vascular anastomoses are completed.

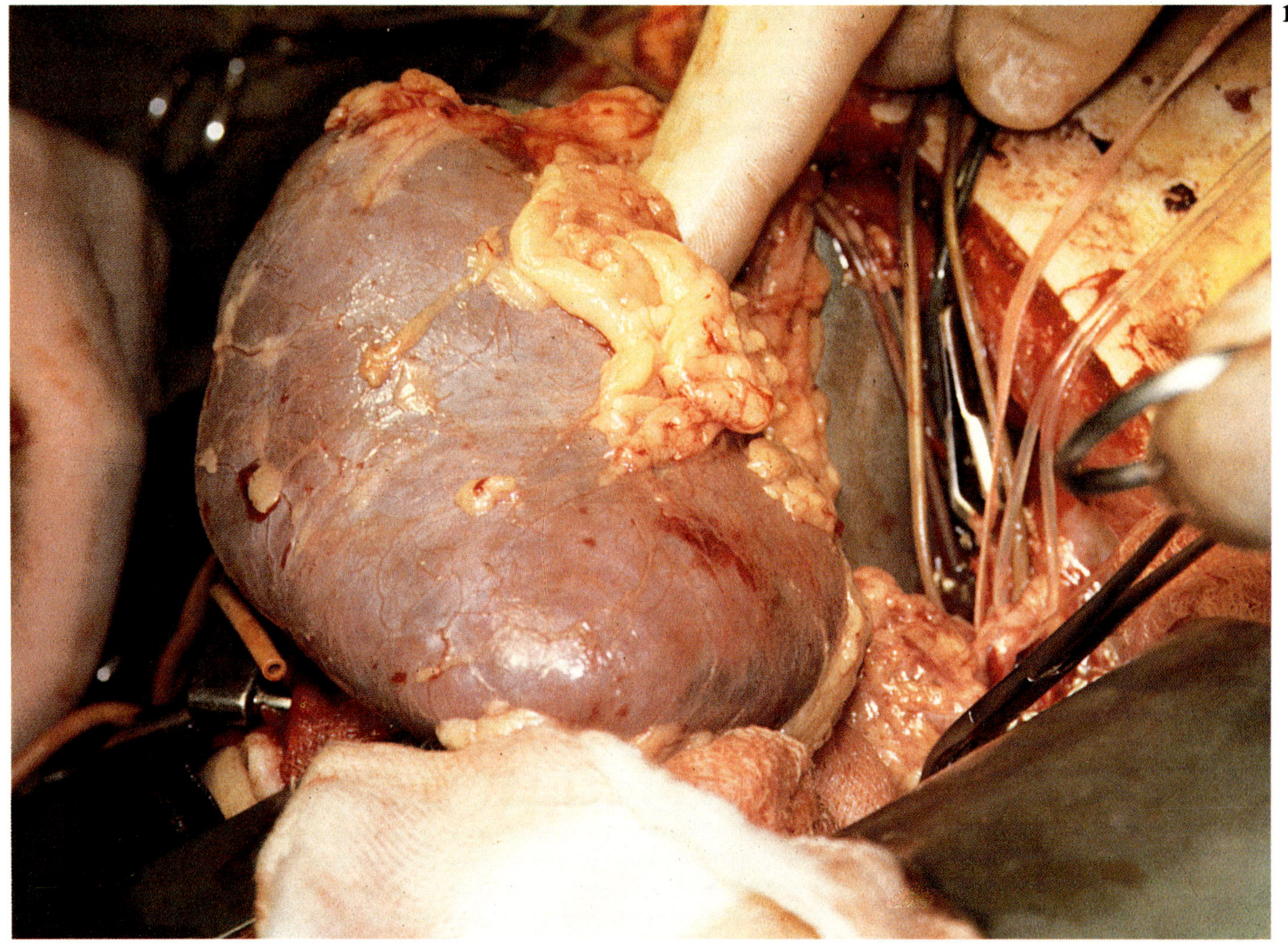

109 Clamps have been taken off the vessels and the kidney has taken on a satisfactory pink colour. The capsular vessels are bleeding.

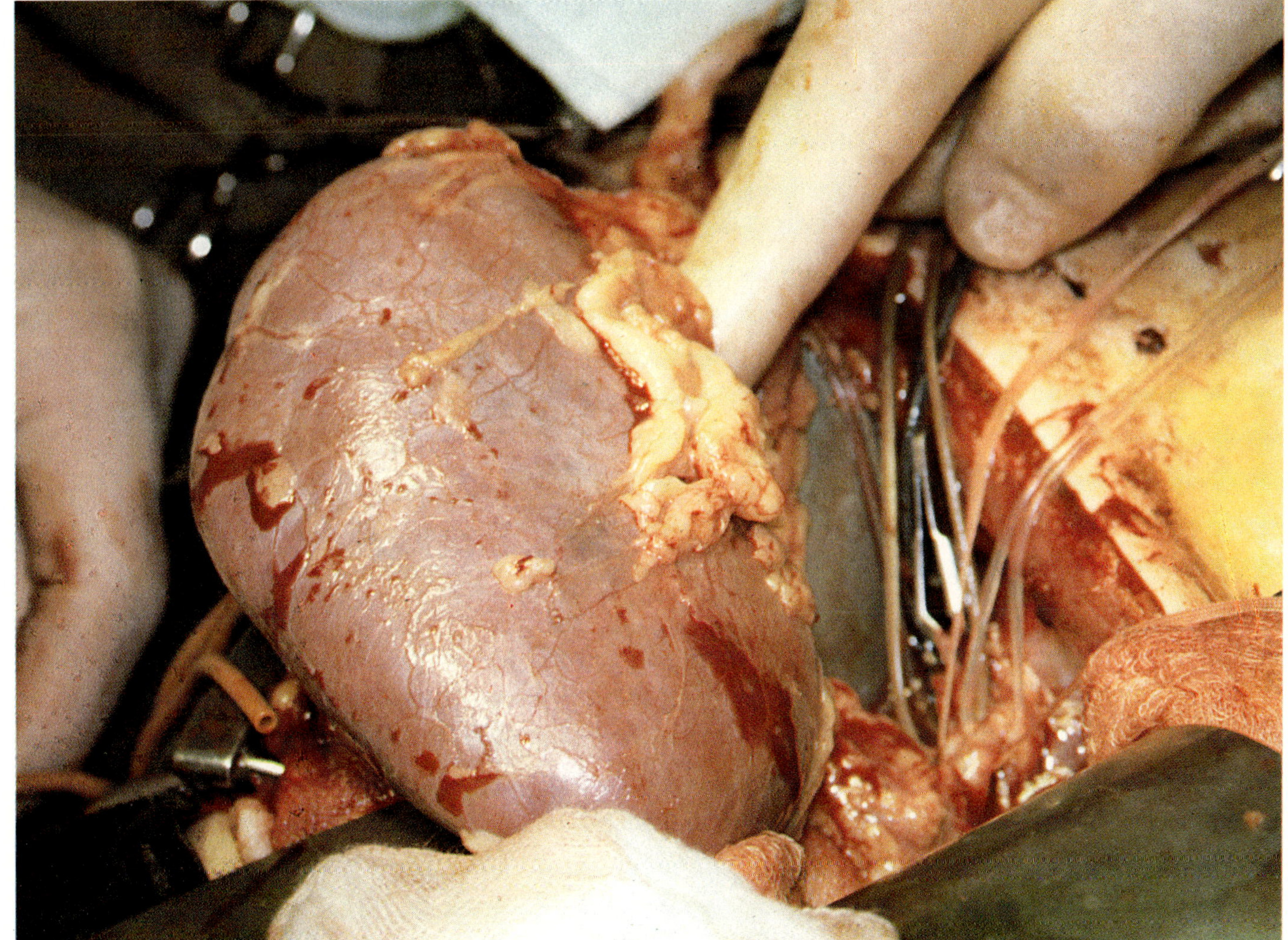

110 An incision has been made in the anterior wall of the bladder on the right side, and the mucosa is pouting.

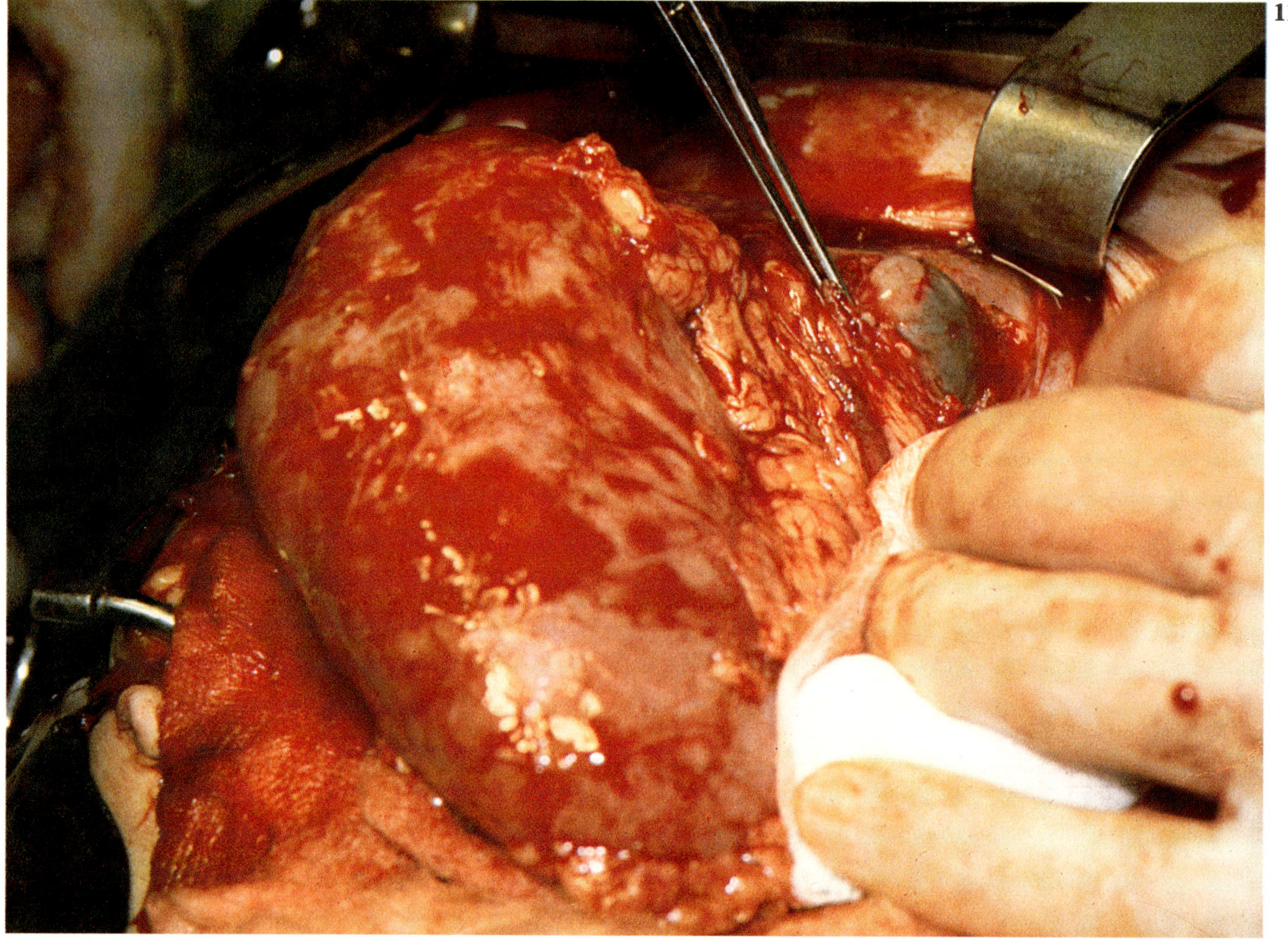

111 **A No. 6 Tizzard catheter has been passed through the bladder wall** and via the incision in the bladder mucosa. The spatulated end of the ureter is being anastomosed to the bladder mucosa.

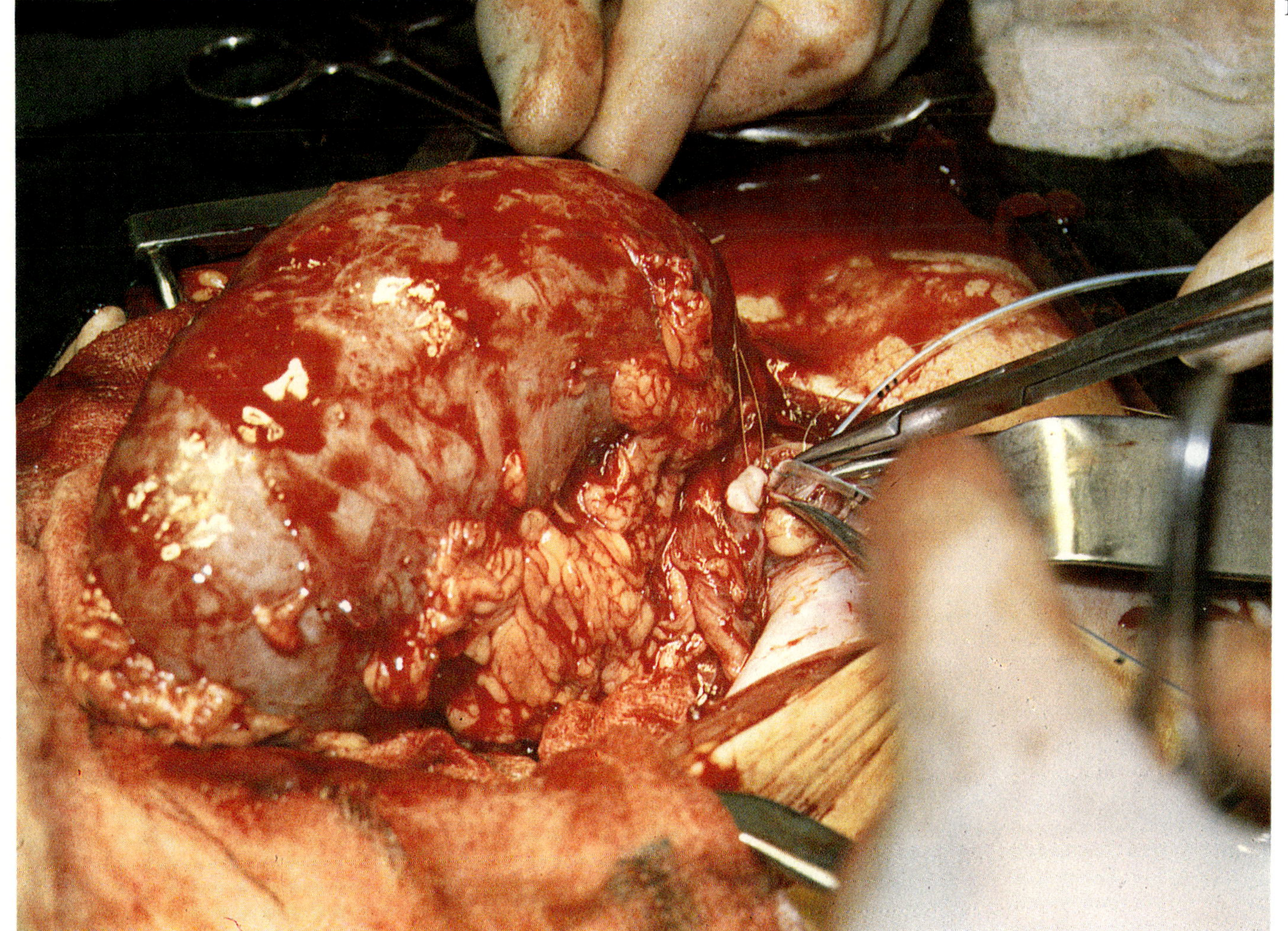

112 The Tizzard catheter is being passed up the ureter.

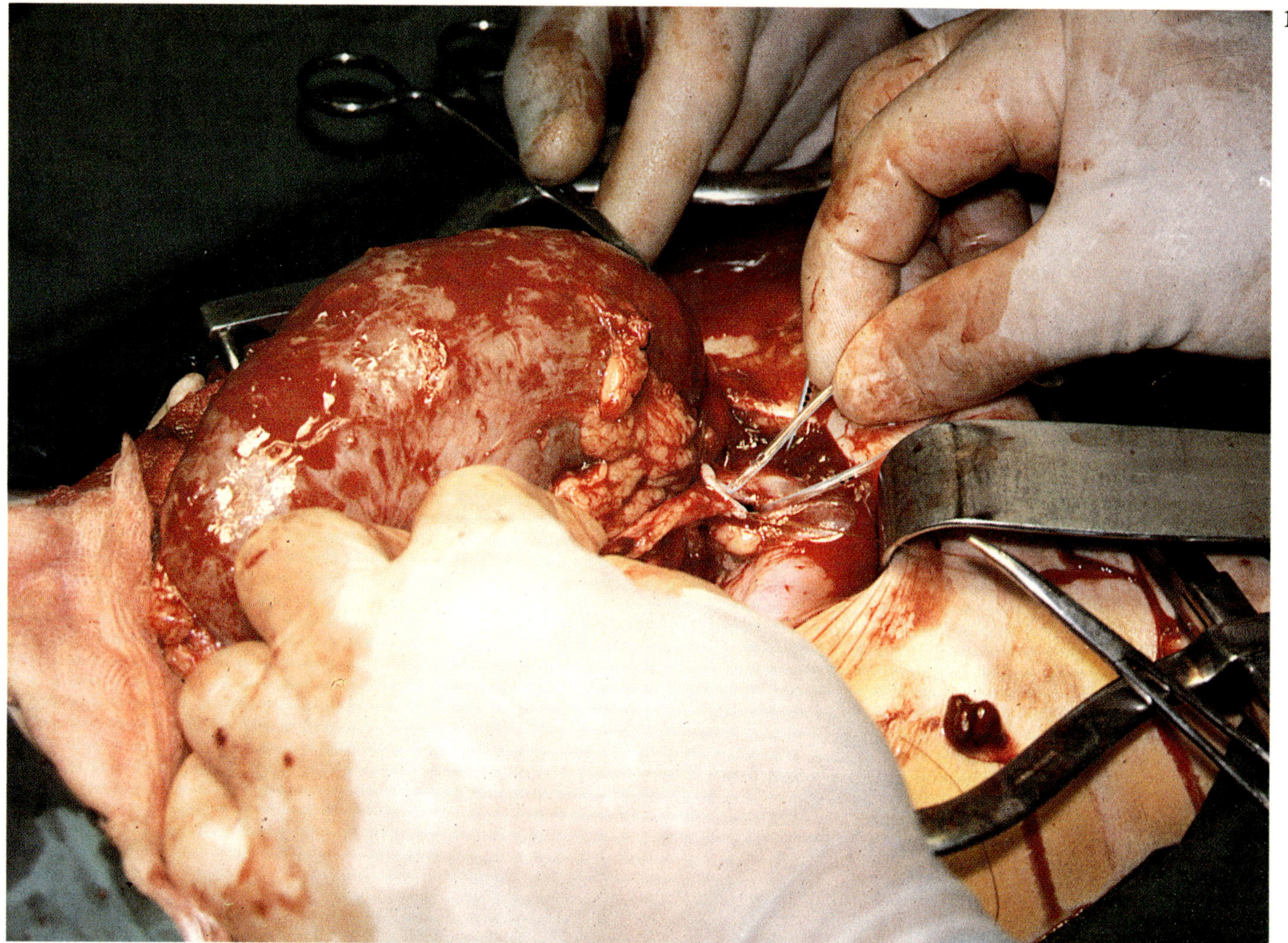

113 The dissected muscle of the bladder is now lifted up and a pair of Moynihan forceps placed in front of the ureter to remain there while the stitches are inserted, so as to prevent too tight a tunnel.

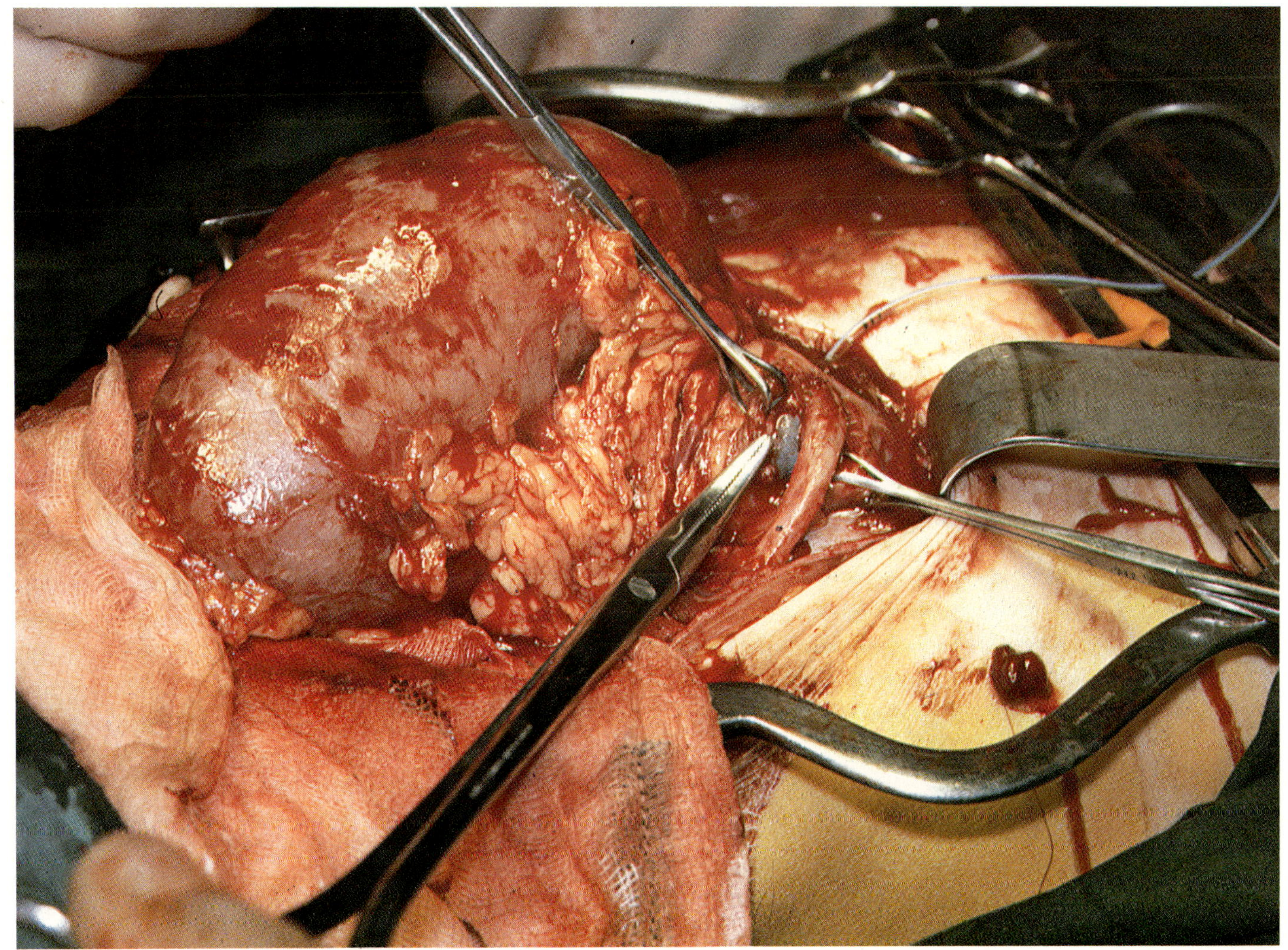

114 The tunnel is about to be constructed.

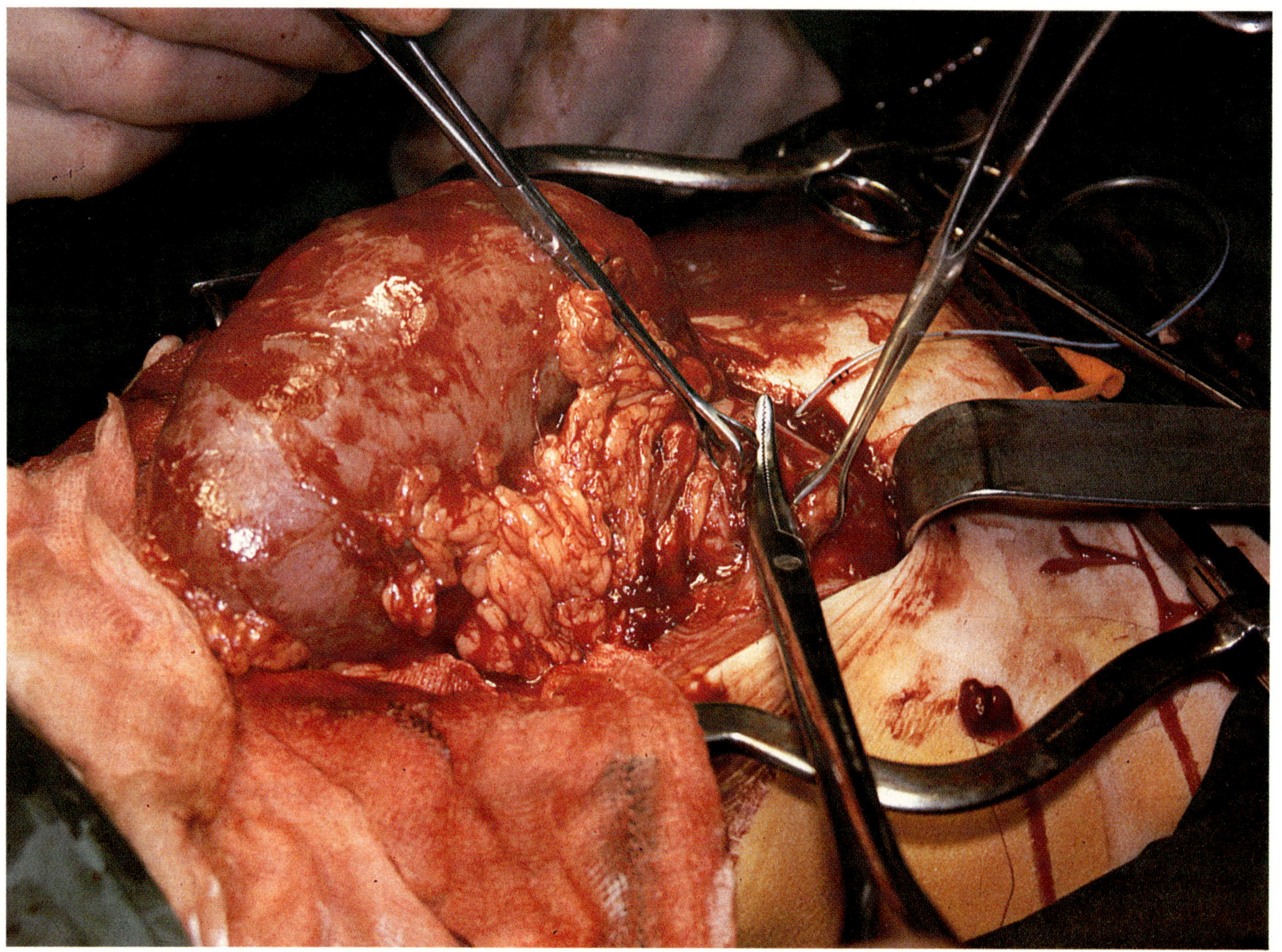

115 The tunnel is now nearly completed and the Moynihan forceps remain in place. Urine can be seen coming out of the Tizzard catheter.

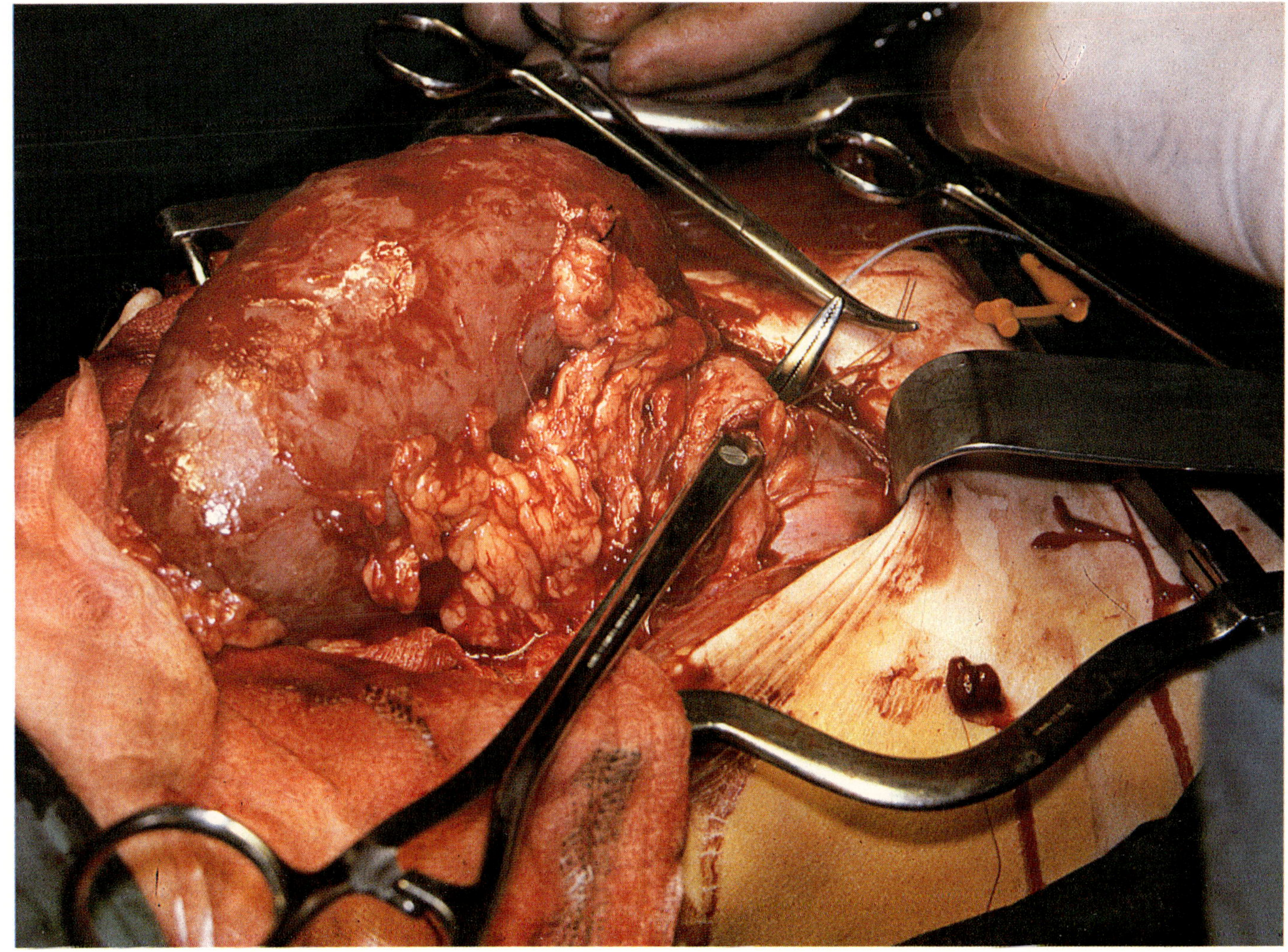

116 Three 2/0 chromic catgut stitches are used to construct the tunnel.

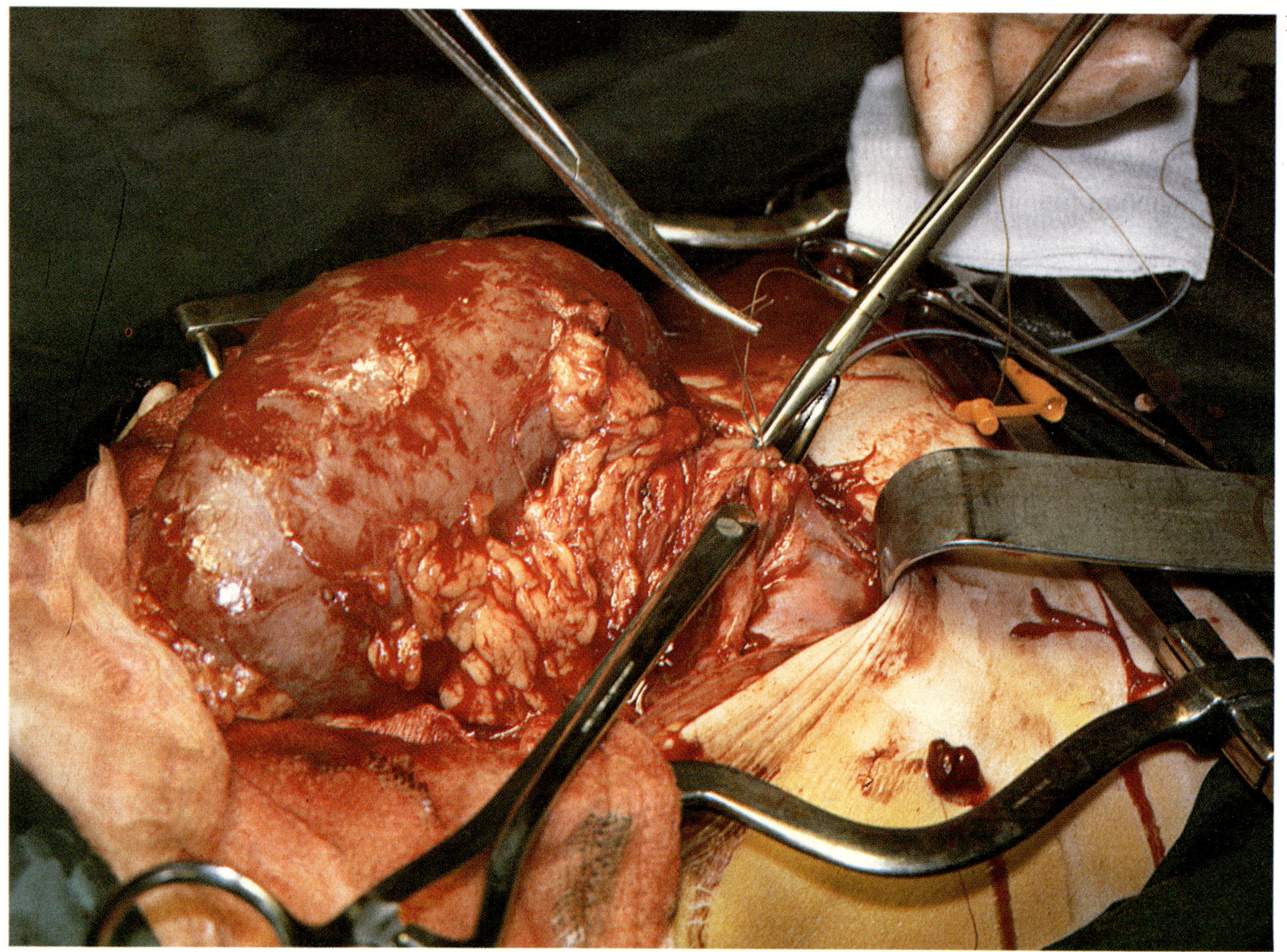

117 The tunnel is now completed. The kidney is fully revascularised and looks satisfactory.

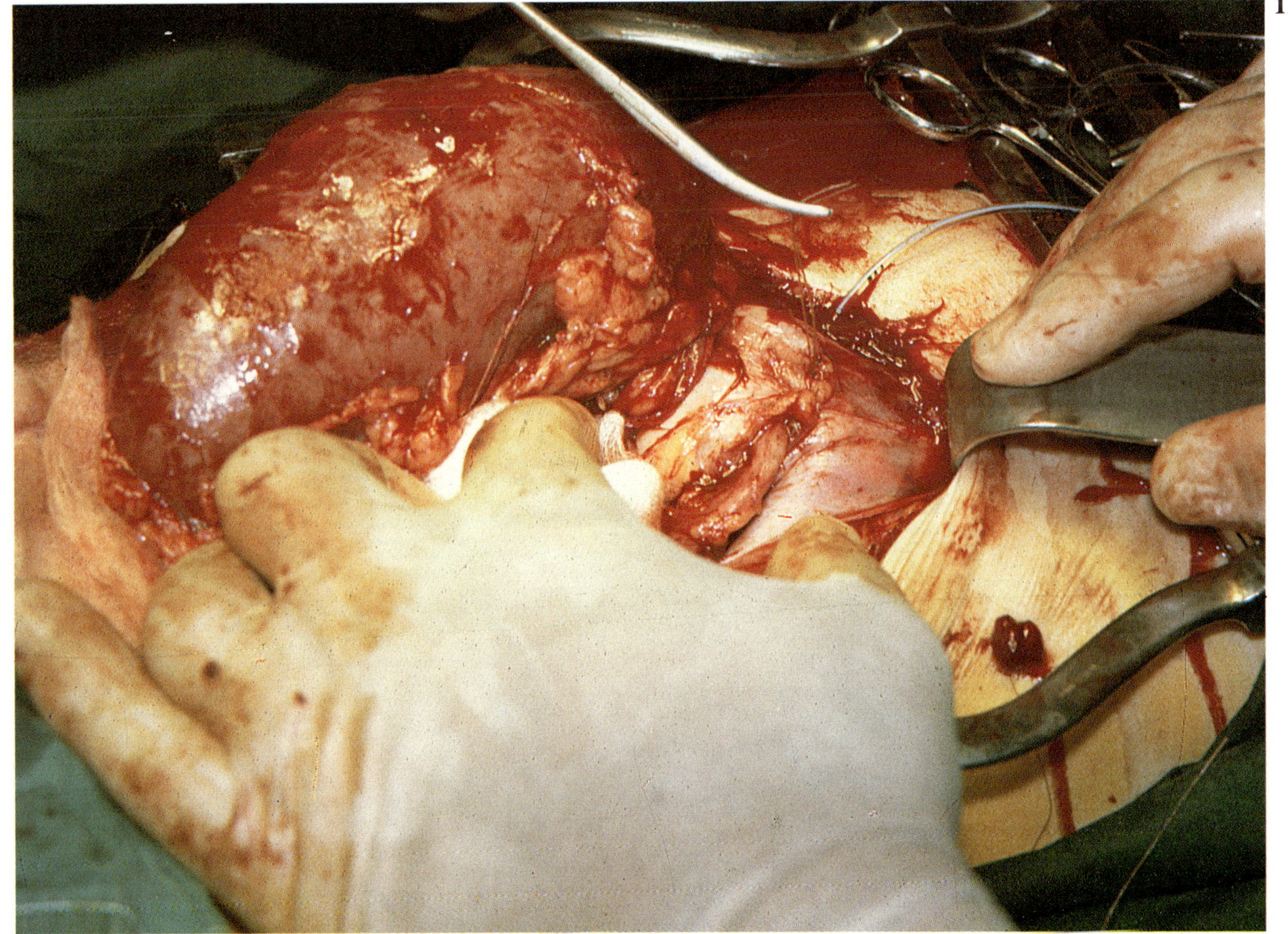

118 The Tizzard catheter has been brought out through a stab incision to the left and below the main wound.

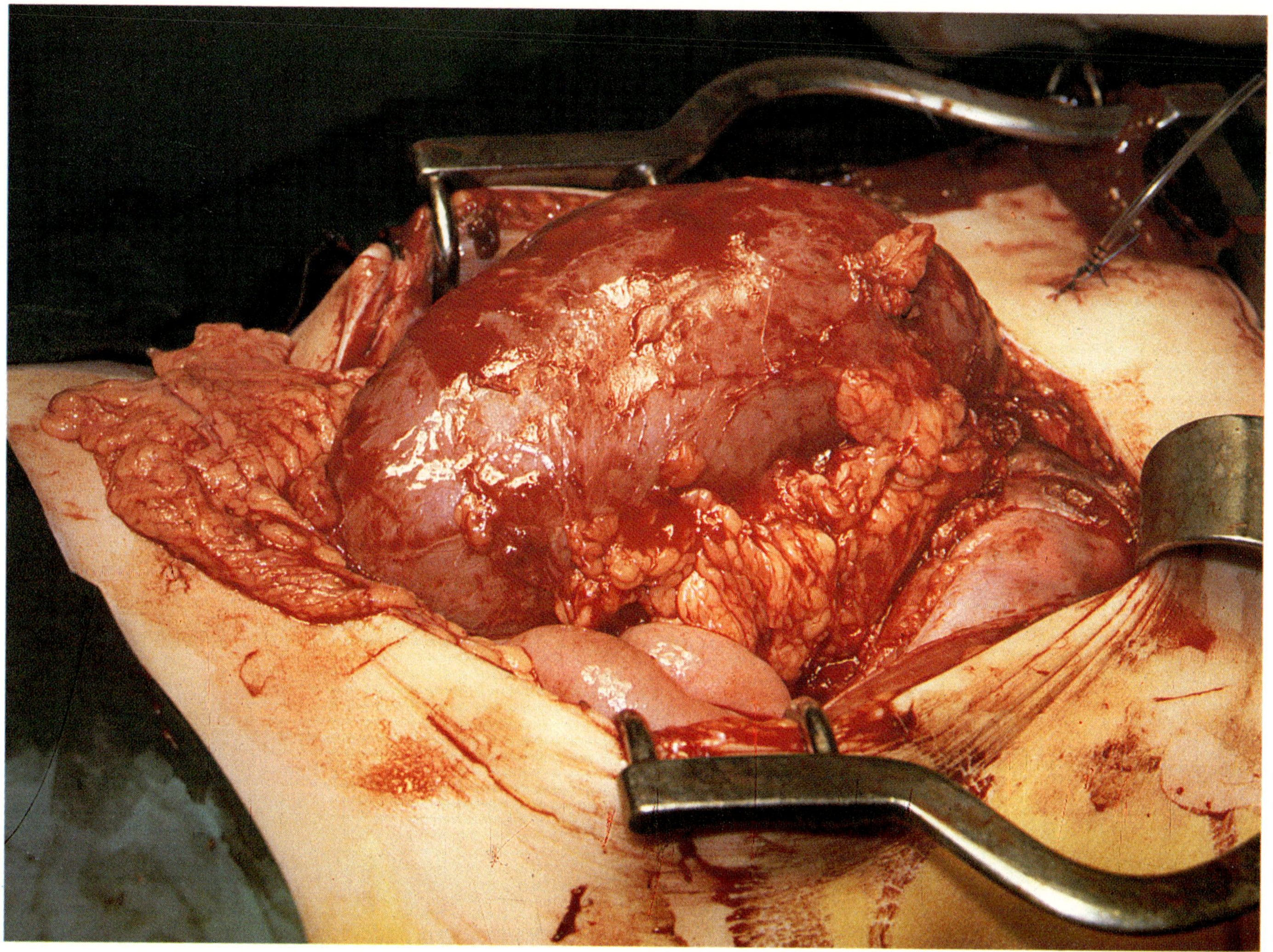

119 The omentum is lifted up and placed over the kidney to protect it from adhesions to bowel.

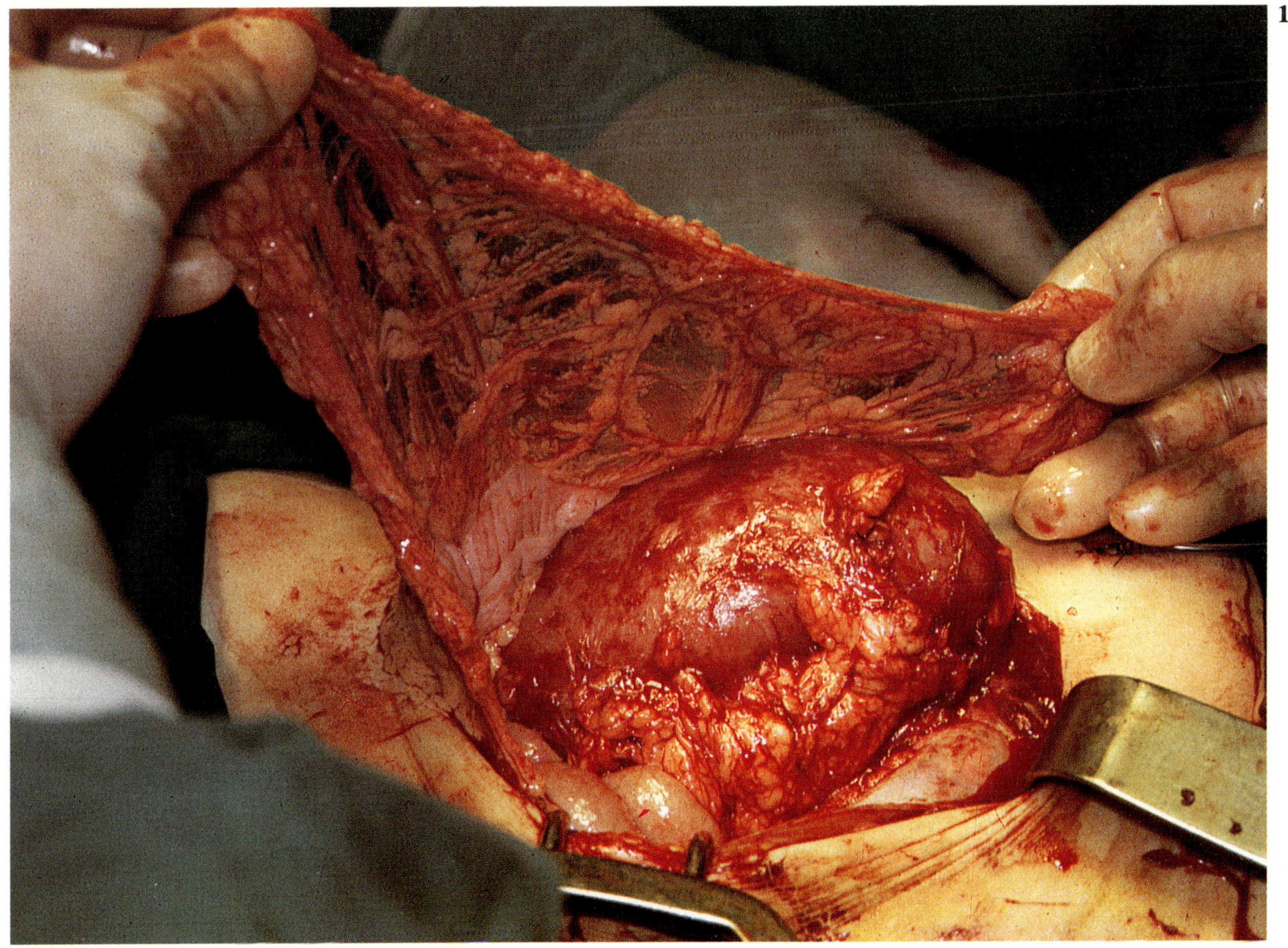

120 **The wound is ready for closure** with continuous looped nylon through all the layers except skin.

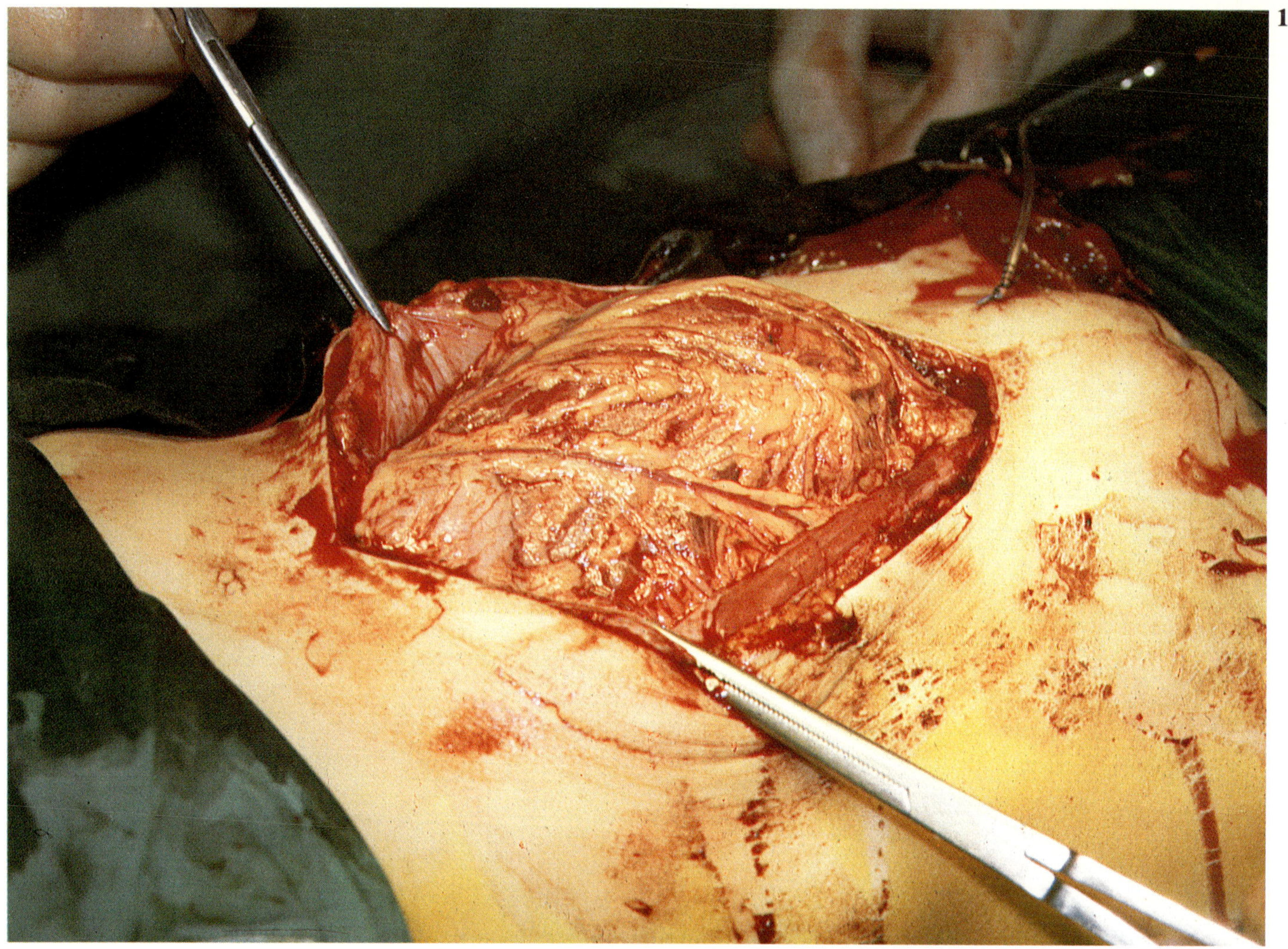

121   Closure in progress.
A 1cm Silastic tube drain
is brought out through a
stab incision in the right
iliac fossa.

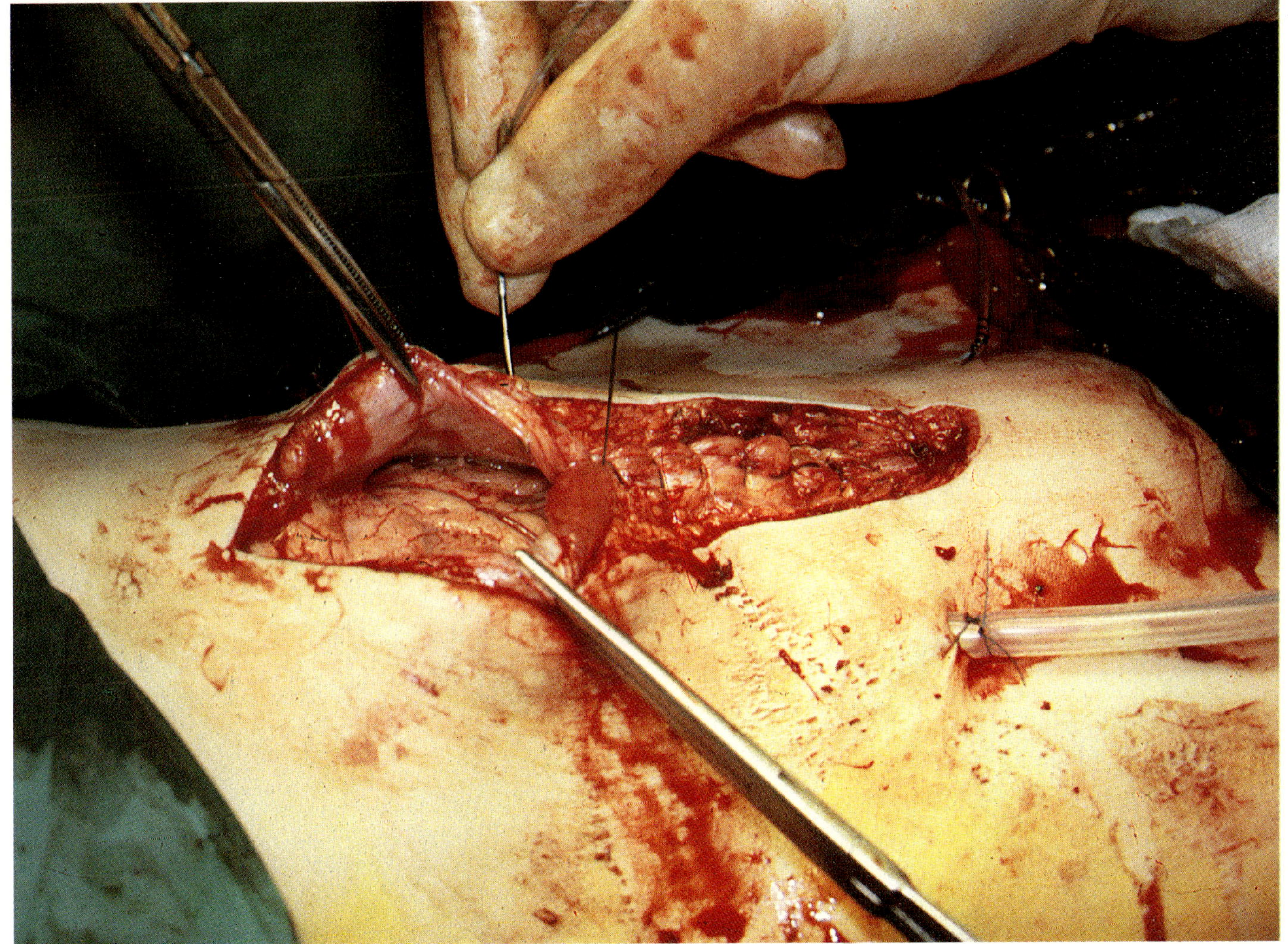

References

[1]*Cadaveric Organs for Transplantation.* A Code of Practice including the Diagnosis of Brain Death. DHSS Health Publications Unit, Heywood, Lancs, 1983.

[2]Pallis, C., 'ABC of Brain-Stem Death'. *British Medical Journal,* London, 1983. (This is a series of articles now available in book form.)

Index

All figures indicate page numbers.